Amazing Diabetes Breakthroughs

Natural Remedies and Medical Miracles That Really Work

Publisher's Note

The editors of FC&A have taken careful measures to ensure the accuracy and usefulness of the information in this book. While every attempt was made to assure accuracy, some Web sites, addresses, telephone numbers, and other information may have changed since printing.

This book is intended for general information only. It does not constitute medical advice or practice. We cannot guarantee the safety or effectiveness of any treatment or advice mentioned. Readers are urged to consult with their health care professionals and get their approval before undertaking therapies suggested by information in this book, keeping in mind that errors in the text may occur as in all publications and that new findings may supercede older information.

> *"Give yourselves to God....Surrender your whole being to him to be used for righteous purposes."*

> *Romans 6:13*

Contents

Blood Sugar Basics

Key answers to your diabetes questions

What is diabetes?

Diabetes is a chronic disease in which you build up too much sugar in your bloodstream. Blood sugar, which scientists call glucose, isn't bad all by itself. In fact, many of your cells need blood sugar for fuel, just like a car needs gasoline to run. But too much of it raises the risk of many health problems. Fortunately, medications, monitoring your blood sugar, and changes to your diet and lifestyle may help delay or avoid these problems.

Diabetes has been around since the days of ancient Egypt, but it got its name from an early Greek physician. The word diabetes comes from a Greek term for siphon, a tube that drains liquid. The Greek physician probably chose this term because frequent urination is a key symptom of diabetes. In fact, doctors later realized that the extra urinating was the body's attempt to get rid of excess blood sugar. That may be why they began calling the condition *diabetes mellitus*. Mellitus, a Latin term meaning "sweet," referred to the high sugar content found in the urine of people with diabetes.

Today more than 20 million people have diabetes. That's around 7 percent of all Americans or about one out of every 15 people. But all diabetes cases aren't the same. Type 1 diabetes mainly affects young people whereas type 2 is more likely to show up in older adults. Here are the basic differences.

▸ Type 1 diabetes is an autoimmune disease. It develops when your immune system gets confused and destroys cells that make insulin, the substance that helps keep your blood sugar from rising too high. This condition also has been called insulin-dependent diabetes because people who have it must have insulin from daily injections or a pump to keep their blood sugar from raging out of control.

▸ Type 2 diabetes occurs when you can't make enough insulin or when your body has lost the ability to use insulin. This is the most common kind of diabetes, especially for adults over age 40. Type 2 diabetes is also called non-insulin dependent diabetes because most people who have it can control their blood sugar without insulin injections.

How common is type 2 diabetes? Who gets it?

At least 90 percent of people with diabetes have type 2 diabetes. That's more than 18 million people, and some experts suggest the true tally may be even higher. What's more, about one out of every five people over age 60 has diabetes, and most of them have type 2. In fact, experts point out that you're more likely to get diabetes after age 40. That's why type 2 is sometimes called maturity onset diabetes.

The good news is that type 2 diabetes is generally milder and easier to control than type 1 diabetes. People with type 1 need insulin shots, but most people with type 2 diabetes can control their blood sugar through weight loss, exercise, dietary changes, and prescription medication.

Where does blood sugar come from?

Your liver makes some of your blood sugar, but you get the rest from foods you eat. During digestion, your body breaks down these foods into basics like sugars and amino acids — and then dumps them into the bloodstream. That's where the sugars become blood sugar.

Your body has a system that makes sure you don't end up with too much blood sugar. Here's how it works. If your blood sugar begins to rise too high, beta cells in your pancreas start pumping out insulin. That insulin signals the liver to stop making blood sugar, so your blood sugar overload won't get worse.

Meanwhile insulin also acts as an "express pass" to quickly move blood sugar out of your bloodstream and into your muscle and liver cells. This not only lowers the sugar levels in your blood, but also delivers fuel (blood sugar) to your liver and muscles. You use some of it immediately, and your body puts the rest in storage.

Insulin also keeps your liver from loading too much sugar into your blood between meals. But if your between-meal blood sugar dips too low, alpha cells in your pancreas release hormones that signal your liver to start making blood sugar again.

Normally these processes are all you need to control blood sugar, but that may change if you get diabetes.

Type 1: not just for kids anymore

Conventional wisdom says that only children develop type 1 diabetes while type 2 pops up solely in adults. But those lines are blurring. Not only are more children and teenagers developing type 2, but scientists have also discovered Latent Autoimmune Diabetes of Adulthood (LADA), a kind of type 1 diabetes that emerges in adults.

LADA initially looks and feels like type 2 diabetes, probably because people with this condition start out with a few beta cells that can still make insulin. When those cells lose that ability, people with LADA need more rigorous medical treatment than those with type 2 diabetes.

Research suggests up to 10 percent of people with type 2 diabetes may have LADA instead. So if you have been diagnosed with type 2, but have difficulty controlling your blood sugar — even after weight loss and medication — ask your doctor about getting tested for LADA.

Why do people with diabetes have too much sugar?

To control blood sugar, your body must do two things. It has to make its own insulin, and it must have the power to use that insulin. People with diabetes have trouble doing one or both of these.

If you have diabetes, the insulin-producing cells in your pancreas may be damaged or destroyed. As a result, either you can't make enough insulin to meet your body's needs or you can no longer produce insulin at all. Without enough insulin, you can't put the brakes on high blood sugar. This happens for two reasons.

▶ You don't have the insulin needed to order your liver to stop making blood sugar.

▶ Your lack of insulin prevents you from moving excess blood sugar out of your blood and into your muscle and liver cells.

Even if you can still produce insulin, you may have trouble controlling your blood sugar thanks to something called insulin resistance. Insulin resistance means your cells don't accept insulin the way they once did. It's almost as if the cells mark the insulin "return to sender."

This triggers a chain reaction that's bad for your health. Because insulin can't get into your muscle and liver cells, it can't give your blood sugar that "express pass" into those cells either. So the next time you get too much blood sugar in your bloodstream, you can't offload it into your muscle and liver cells fast enough. Without this valuable safety valve, your blood sugar can build up to dangerous levels.

How does insulin resistance relate to diabetes?

Insulin resistance is the first and mildest stage of type 2 diabetes. Research suggests you may have the power to determine whether it gets worse or better over time. Remember, insulin resistance means blood sugar may not get into your muscle and liver cells because those cells are losing their ability to accept it. But that doesn't mean the cells never let insulin in. If the beta cells in your pancreas churn out a lot more insulin than usual, the resulting flood of insulin can overcome insulin resistance. Once this happens, your blood sugar can zip into the cells so the amount of sugar in your bloodstream drops.

But over time, your overworked beta cells lose their ability to produce torrents of insulin. When that happens, you start having blood sugar overloads immediately after meals, and those cause damage in your body. Eventually, high blood sugar begins to injure and destroy beta cells in your pancreas. They gradually produce less and less insulin until you can't make your own insulin anymore. Then your blood sugar levels stay high most of the time, and you need insulin shots to survive.

Clearly, insulin resistance can lead to a worst-case scenario, but you have the chance to prevent that by changing your diet. Some research suggests that eating high-sugar foods and refined carbohydrates like white bread may contribute to insulin resistance. So if you eat those foods constantly, you may be tempting fate. But research also suggests hearty whole grains and other high-fiber foods help improve your body's ability to use insulin. Try trading sugary items and refined carbohydrates for foods packed with fiber. You may be pleasantly surprised at the results.

What is prediabetes? Is it the same as syndrome X?

These two health menaces are not the same, but they are related. Think of prediabetes as just one ingredient in the recipe for syndrome X. But you can be prediabetic even if you don't have the more complicated syndrome. Here are the two conditions in a nutshell.

Prediabetes. You're four times more likely to have a fatal heart attack if you have high blood sugar. Yet doctors often don't treat it or even explain it. Here are the lifesaving facts you should know.

Prediabetes means your blood sugar is higher than normal, but not yet high enough for the full danger of diabetes. If your doctor says your blood sugar is between 100-125 milligrams per deciliter (mg/dL), you have prediabetes. Don't ignore a diagnosis of high-normal blood sugar – it's more dangerous than it sounds. It means you're likely to develop full-blown diabetes within 10 years unless you make diabetes-fighting lifestyle changes or take medication. Fortunately, exercise and weight loss can substantially lower your odds of turning prediabetes into type 2 diabetes.

Syndrome X. More commonly known as metabolic syndrome, this is a combination of symptoms that puts you at high risk for diabetes, heart disease, and stroke. The symptoms are prediabetes or diabetes, high blood pressure, low levels of "good" HDL cholesterol, high triglycerides in your blood, and obesity where fat accumulates around your midsection. Up to 25 percent of Americans may have this dangerous condition. If you think you have any one of these symptoms, ask your doctor about metabolic syndrome. He can find out whether you have it and help you take steps to protect yourself from the devastating consequences.

What is the major risk factor for diabetes?

Obesity helps fuel both insulin resistance and type 2 diabetes – especially if your extra weight is mostly around the middle and upper parts of your body. Why? Adding fat cells makes all your body cells more stubbornly resistant to insulin. So the more you weigh, the higher your risk of diabetes soars. That's why obesity is the leading risk factor for diabetes. It's also why doctors encourage people with early warning signs of diabetes to lose weight, change their eating habits, and take up exercise.

If you're not sure whether you're obese, just grab a tape measure and wrap it around your waist. A waist size of 35 inches or more for women or 40 inches or more for men is considered obese.

What are other risk factors for diabetes?

A new study suggests that 73 million Americans either have diabetes or are at risk of developing it. The more of these that apply to you, the higher your risk of type 2 diabetes may be.

▸ You have at least one relative with diabetes.

▸ You are 45 or older.

▸ You are African American, Hispanic, Asian, or Native American.

▸ You are obese. Nearly 80 percent of all people with type 2 diabetes have this problem.

▸ Your extra weight sits mostly around your waist instead of at your hips.

▸ Your doctor says you have metabolic syndrome, which includes problems with blood pressure, cholesterol, triglycerides, and blood sugar in addition to obesity and insulin resistance.

▸ You smoke or are exposed to second-hand smoke.

▸ Your doctor says you have prediabetes, meaning your blood sugar is above normal but not high enough to be diagnosed as diabetes.

▸ You exercise less than three times a week and lead a sedentary life.

▸ You have a disease that damages the pancreas or interferes with your ability to make insulin.

▸ You take thiazide diuretic drugs for blood pressure, corticosteroid medications, or other medications that put you at risk for diabetes. Talk to your doctor about medications that could affect your risk of diabetes or its complications.

▸ You had gestational diabetes during pregnancy or gave birth to a baby that weighed 9 pounds or more.

New research shows that up to half the American population may have a gene that raises the risk of diabetes. So, if you have one of these risk factors and have not been tested for diabetes in the last three years, don't take chances. Ask your doctor whether you need to be screened.

What are the symptoms of diabetes?

You may be one of nearly 6 million Americans who already have diabetes and don't know it. The most common signs of diabetes are seemingly harmless symptoms like more frequent urination than usual, increased thirst and appetite, and drinking extra fluids. Other symptoms may include these:

▶ tiredness and weakness

▶ gum infections, bleeding gums, or skin infections

▶ weight changes such as weight loss

▶ vision changes such as blurred vision

▶ repeated vaginal yeast infections in women or erectile dysfunction in men

▶ tingling or burning in your fingers, toes, arms, or legs

How do you know if you have diabetes?

Up to half of all people with diabetes either don't show symptoms or haven't noticed their symptoms. Perhaps that's why the American Diabetes Association recommends diabetes screening if you are age 45 or older. They also recommend screening if you are under 45 but have other risk factors for diabetes. Getting screened isn't much harder than taking a blood test. And, fortunately, it's never too late to stop – even reverse – the harmful effects of type 2 diabetes. Here's what you can expect from screening tests.

Casual plasma glucose test. This is just a regular blood test. Once the nurse draws a little blood sample from you, the lab tallies your blood sugar. Your doctor may suggest this test if you've already shown classic symptoms of diabetes like excessive thirst or mysterious weight loss. If your sugar level is 200 milligrams per deciliter (mg/dL) or more, you probably have diabetes.

Fasting plasma glucose test (FPG). This blood test measures your blood sugar levels after you've avoided food for eight hours. Although doctors consider this the best test for accurately diagnosing diabetes, your doctor may ask you to take it twice to be certain the results are correct. If both tests find a blood sugar level of 126 mg/dL or higher, you probably have diabetes.

Oral glucose tolerance test. To take this test, you avoid food for eight hours and then drink a specially prescribed beverage with a high glucose (sugar) content. Two hours later, a nurse draws a sample of your blood to check your blood sugar. A level of 200 mg/dL or more indicates diabetes, while 140 to 199 mg/dL suggests prediabetes. Your doctor may recommend this test if your FPG appeared normal, but you still have symptoms or risk factors

Testing cuts health dangers

Diabetes raises your risk of complications like vision loss, amputation, kidney failure, and heart attacks, but a simple blood test may help you fight back. It's called the Hemoglobin A1c (HbA1c) test, and it shows your true average level of blood sugar over the previous few months. Doctors routinely give the HbA1c test about every three months.

A result of more than 7 percent or 170 mg/dL means you're at high risk for complications. If you're not already monitoring your blood sugar level at home at least once a day, you should start. Research suggests extra monitoring and stricter control can help cut your risk of disabling health problems.

for diabetes. But be aware this test is also more likely to find evidence for diabetes when you don't really have it.

What complications may develop from untreated diabetes?

Diabetes may start by wreaking havoc with your blood sugar, but the trouble doesn't stop there. All that extra blood sugar gradually damages other parts of your body over time. That's why it leads to complications like these.

Vision loss. High blood sugar can damage small blood vessels in your retina. This can lead to diabetic retinopathy, blurred vision, and blindness. In addition, diabetes raises your odds of cataracts and glaucoma. So it's no wonder diabetes is the leading cause of blindness in adults aged 20 to 74.

Heart disease, heart attack, and stroke. People with diabetes are two to four times more likely to die of stroke. Adults with diabetes are also far more likely to die of heart disease.

Nerve damage. At least 60 percent of people with diabetes have neuropathy (nerve damage). This can lead to pain or impaired feeling in your hands or feet, slowed digestion in your stomach, carpal tunnel syndrome, and, in severe cases, foot amputation.

Foot problems. People with diabetes are more likely to develop peripheral arterial disease, a condition that hampers the blood flow to your feet. Diabetes may also lead to nerve damage in your feet. Together, these limitations make foot problems, such as infection, more dangerous. Low blood flow may prevent foot damage from healing properly while nerve damage keeps some people from catching the problem before amputation becomes necessary. That's why careful foot care is so important.

Dental disease. Periodontal gum disease is more likely if you have diabetes. It starts with bleeding, swelling, and tenderness in the gums, but it can lead to tooth loss.

Kidney disease. Diabetes is the leading cause of kidney disease. Thousands of people with diabetes already suffer from this condition.

Parkinson's disease. New research from Finland suggests people with type 2 diabetes may have a higher risk of developing Parkinson's disease.

A new report suggests that complications like these can cost each person with diabetes up to $10,000 a year, including $1,600 in out-of-pocket costs. Fortunately, lifestyle changes, smart eating choices, and savvy new health habits can help blunt or prevent these problems.

How is diabetes related to other conditions?

Experts believe diabetes and other conditions like cancer, heart problems, and bowel disease may be tied together by one hidden factor – inflammation. They have found that inflammation has a link to every one of these conditions, plus high blood pressure, arthritis, weight control, and more. But knowing how inflammation begins can help you fight back.

Inflammation is your immune system's normal quick response to threats like infection or injury. White blood cells rush to the scene and release chemicals to fight the intruder. The resulting inflammation restores order and protects you. But sometimes these powerful immune cells overdo it. Then the inflammation – marked by redness, heat, swelling, and pain – becomes a bigger problem than the original threat.

Your immune system can also run amok and unleash its inflammatory chemicals on normal tissue. That's what happens in autoimmune disorders like rheumatoid arthritis. In obese people, fat cells produce compounds that promote inflammation. Research suggests this inflammation contributes to insulin resistance. That's a key reason why weight loss helps fight diabetes.

Here are some of the other conditions that may result from inflammation.

▶ **Heart attack and stroke.** Experts now believe inflammation plays a major role in these events. In fact, higher levels of C-reactive protein, a sign of inflammation, mean a higher risk for heart attack, high blood pressure, and stroke.

▶ **Cancer.** Inflammation may interfere with normal cell death and produce DNA-damaging free radicals, leading to cancer. Normal inflammatory processes may even help the cancer spread.

▶ **Gastrointestinal problems.** Inflammatory bowel disease, which includes Crohn's disease and colitis, can wreak havoc with your whole digestive system. Even ulcers stem from inflammation triggered by a bacterial infection.

▶ **Alzheimer's disease.** Research suggests exposure to inflammation may raise the risk of Alzheimer's while anti-inflammatory drugs like aspirin and ibuprofen may help reduce that risk.

Common treatments for inflammation involve anti-inflammatory drugs, including statins, aspirin, and ibuprofen. But you can also reduce inflammation through diet and weight loss. For more information, see the chapters *Diet Defense: Smart eating to balance blood sugar,* and *Slimming Down: Simple steps to reverse diabetes.*

What steps can you take to avoid type 2 diabetes or its complications?

Diabetes puts you at risk for possible blindness, amputation, and heart failure. If you're over age 45 or have heart disease or diabetes in the family, don't wait to take action. According to a new report, the cost of treating diabetes in America is around $37 billion a year. But that figure skyrockets to $57 billion when people develop complications because they didn't follow their doctor's diet, exercise, and medication advice.

Fortunately, you can prevent diabetes with only modest changes in weight and activity, even if you have high blood sugar. In fact, you can stop diabetes in its tracks with three simple steps. No drugs, no starvation diets, no kidding. Just control your blood sugar naturally with these essential tips.

Choose lifestyle changes over drugs. A groundbreaking research study suggests drugs are much less beneficial than natural methods of control. The researchers recruited people who were overweight and had high blood sugar, but didn't have diabetes. One group in the study exercised and lost weight while the other group took the diabetes drug metformin (Glucophage). Although the drug group cut their risk of diabetes by 31 percent, the exercise and weight loss group cut their diabetes risk by nearly 60 percent without drugs.

The study participants did just 30 minutes of moderate exercise – like walking – five days a week. They also lost 15 pounds through a low-fat diet. This combination of exercise and weight loss also lowers your risk of heart disease and stroke.

Other lifestyle changes will also help you beat diabetes. For example, smoking raises your risk of heart trouble and foot-threatening nerve damage and blood-flow problems. Quitting could cut your risk of heart attack, stroke, and amputation.

Trade bad carbs for good carbs. Make the switch from refined carbohydrates like sugary foods to high-fiber carbohydrates. For example, instead of a sugary-sweet breakfast cereal, try a low-sugar, high-fiber cereal. Research suggests women can cut their diabetes risk by more than a third this way. You might also lower your heart attack risk and avoid blood flow problems that endanger your feet. Learn more about smart carb choices in *The Glycemic Index* chapter.

Stop eating the wrong fats. Avoid trans fats, and cut back on saturated fats like meats, high-fat dairy products, and butter. Instead, eat fish rich in omega-3 fats like sardines twice a week. You can also enjoy limited amounts of other "good" fats like avocados, olive oil, and nuts.

The Glycemic Index

How to take control of your blood sugar

What is the glycemic index?

Your body burns sugar like your car burns gas, and carbohydrates are your main source of this fuel. Different carbs break down into glucose – or sugar – at different rates, depending on their structure. Some burn quickly, releasing a flood of glucose into your bloodstream. To counter that, your body needs to release a large amount of insulin. Other carbohydrates take longer to digest, giving you a slower, steadier supply of glucose.

The glycemic index (GI) measures a food's ability to raise your blood sugar. Foods that burn faster have a higher GI value, while slower-burning foods have a low one. Just as the slow and steady tortoise beat the speedy hare in the famous fable, the slow-burning carbohydrates have the advantage when it comes to your health. They keep your insulin, your blood sugar, and your appetite steady.

The glycemic index is a valuable tool if you need to control your blood sugar levels. Rather than lump all carbohydrates together and avoid or severely restrict them all, you can make smart decisions based on a food's GI. As you'll discover, using the glycemic index can help you control your diabetes, lose weight, and enjoy mealtimes.

Master the mystery of the GI value

Researchers, like Dr. Jennie Brand-Miller and colleagues at the University of Sydney in Australia, determine GI values of foods through rigorous testing. Here's how it works.

After an overnight fast, a group of at least 10 volunteers eats 50 grams of available carbohydrate of the test food. Using blood samples taken at frequent intervals over the next two hours, researchers plot the volunteers' blood sugar response on a curve. They calculate the area under the curve (AUC) to determine the total rise in blood sugar.

Then they go through the same process with a reference food, either pure glucose or white bread. Dividing the AUC of the test food by the AUC of the reference food and multiplying by 100 gives you the GI value of the test food. The average GI rating of all 10 or more volunteers becomes the GI value for the test food.

As the reference food, glucose has a GI of 100. The GI values of other foods are expressed as percentages of the effect of glucose. For example, a dinner roll has a GI of 73, so the rise in blood sugar after eating a dinner roll is 73 percent as great as after eating pure glucose.

Foods with a GI of 70 or higher are considered high-GI foods. Foods in the 56-69 range are medium or moderate, while those with a GI of 55 or less are low-GI foods.

So far, more than 500 foods have been tested. You can find published lists of these foods in books – including this one – or online. The glycemic index technically applies only to carbohydrates because fats and proteins do not have the same effect on blood sugar. But several common foods with no measurable carbohydrates, like meats

GI reference food standardized

When the glycemic index was developed at the University of Toronto in 1981, scientists used a 50-gram portion of white bread as the standard of measurement. But some foods raise blood glucose higher than white bread's value of 100. When the glucose = 100 scale was implemented, white bread was determined to have a value of only 70. Although you may still see references to the white-bread scale, the use of two standards has become confusing, and the glucose scale is now recommended.

and some vegetables, also appear on these lists to give you a wider range of options.

Fuel your body with the right carbs

Lately, "carb" has become a four-letter word. Popular diets, like the Atkins Diet, severely restrict carbohydrates as a way to promote weight loss. While you may lose weight by cutting out carbohydrates, you'll also lose your body's main source of energy and brainpower. You'll also lose many natural sources of vitamins and minerals, fiber, and water.

Your body needs carbohydrates, which take the form of starches, sugars, and dietary fiber. As you digest carbohydrates, your body converts them to glucose, which it burns for energy. For some foods (those with high GI values), this happens very quickly. For others, it takes a while to break them down.

You find carbohydrates mostly in cereal grains, fruits, starchy vegetables, legumes, and dairy products. The key is to choose the right ones – and that's where the glycemic index can help. In the past, dietary advice for people with diabetes included counting carbohydrates. But that tactic assumes all carbohydrates have the same effect on your blood sugar – a myth debunked by the glycemic index. It's the type of carbohydrate you choose, not the total amount, that makes a difference.

Another myth, involving the distinction between simple and complex carbohydrates, also went up in smoke. The prevailing wisdom was that simple carbohydrates, like sugar, had a greater impact on your blood sugar levels, while complex carbohydrates, like starches, had less of an effect. Surprisingly, GI testing has found that the reverse is often true.

Sugar is actually a moderate GI food, while some starches – like potatoes – cause a rapid spike in blood glucose. It goes to show the importance of testing. It's the only way to know for sure how a food affects your blood sugar levels.

Several factors can affect a food's GI rating. Here is a quick look at some of them.

▸ Type of starch. The more swollen, or gelatinized, a starch becomes, the quicker your body digests it and the higher its glycemic index.

▸ Ripeness. Ripe fruits and vegetables have higher sugar contents, raising their GI values.

▸ Particle size. Finely ground grain is much easier to digest because of its small particle size. Coarsely ground grain, like stone-ground flours, have lower GI rates.

▸ Fiber. Viscous fiber, the soluble kind found in oats, beans, and apples, slows the movement of food through your intestines. This prevents your digestive enzymes from breaking down starches too quickly.

▸ Fat. Fat slows down stomach emptying, so it takes longer to digest starches.

▸ Acidity. Like fats, acids slow down stomach emptying and lead to slower digestion. Vinegar and citrus juices work in this manner.

In general, the more processed a food, the higher its glycemic index. That explains why diabetes has become more of a problem as our diets have changed to include more highly processed foods.

Use glycemic load for maximum results

While useful, the glycemic index alone does not account for portion size. You can choose all low-GI foods, but if you eat too many of them, you will still end up overweight and battling high blood sugar. That's where the glycemic load (GL) comes in.

Glycemic load takes into account both the GI value of a food and portion size to calculate the effect it will have on your blood sugar. Harvard University researchers developed the formula for GL. To figure it out, you need to know the GI value of a food as well as its available carbohydrate content. That means total carbohydrates minus fiber, which your body does not digest. Multiply the GI by the available carbohydrate and divide that number by 100 to get a food's GL.

To understand GL, keep in mind that a food's GL equals grams of glucose. In other words, a food with a GL of 10 has the same effect on your blood sugar as 10 grams of glucose.

A glycemic load of 10 or below is low, between 11 and 19 is medium, and 20 or above is high. If you're trying to lose weight, your total GL for each day should fall between 60 and 75. For extremely active people, this jumps to 100-150.

Some foods with a high GI, like watermelon, actually have a low GL because the available carbohydrate content in a normal serving size is much less than the 50 grams used when testing the food's GI. On the other hand, eating a large portion of a low-GI food, like a huge bowl of pasta, will raise the GL of your meal. Luckily, you don't have to do math before every meal. Many GI lists now also include the food's GL, as well as its standard serving size.

Keep in mind that glycemic load can be misleading. If a food is low in carbohydrates but high in saturated fat, like sausage or bacon, its GL will be low – but it won't be a healthy food choice.

GI: key to managing diabetes

Making food choices based on the glycemic index can have a very beneficial effect on your health – especially if you have diabetes. As you know, controlling your blood sugar levels is key to managing diabetes.

'Free' foods to fill up on

Some foods have no GI value because they have little or no carbohydrates. To test them, volunteers would have to eat an alarming amount of the food to reach 50 grams of available carbohydrate. Consider them "free" foods you can fill up on without hurting your blood sugar. Would you believe nuts are on the list?

- alfalfa sprouts
- artichokes
- arugula
- asparagus
- avocado
- bean sprouts
- broccoli
- Brussels sprouts
- cabbage
- cauliflower
- celery
- chili peppers
- chives
- cucumber
- eggplant
- endive
- fennel
- garlic
- ginger
- green beans
- herbs
- leeks
- lemon
- lettuce
- lime
- mushrooms
- nuts
- okra
- onions
- peppers
- radishes
- raspberries
- rhubarb
- scallions
- shallots
- snow pea sprouts
- spinach
- yellow squash
- Swiss chard
- tomato
- turnip
- watercress
- zucchini

Other foods with no GI — but plenty of protein or fat — include bacon, cheese, ground beef, chicken without skin and bone, steamed clams, fish, ham, lamb, lobster, oysters, pork, salami, salmon, sardines, scallops, shrimp, tuna, turkey, and veal. These foods won't affect your blood sugar, but not all of them are healthy choices. For beverages with no GI, sip black coffee, diet soda, or water.

Eating high-GI foods leads to rapid spikes and plunges in your blood sugar levels. This rollercoaster response puts a heavy burden on your system. You need to use more insulin to handle the flood of glucose. Eventually this leads to insulin resistance, where your body no longer responds to insulin so it takes more and more insulin to achieve the same effect. Insulin resistance plays a role in the development of type 2 diabetes.

On the other hand, opting for low-GI foods leads to a slow, steady release of glucose that's much easier for your body to handle. In fact, simply changing to a low-GI diet may help you control diabetes better than some of the latest expensive diabetes drugs and insulins.

It can also help you sidestep the serious complications associated with diabetes, like leg amputations, blindness, kidney failure, heart attacks, and strokes. That's because high levels of blood glucose damage the blood vessels in the heart, legs, brains, eyes, and kidneys. High levels of insulin may also harm blood vessels. When you eat high-GI foods, your blood vessels get a double dose of trouble − a rush of glucose followed by another rush of insulin. If you switch to a low-GI diet, you can protect your blood vessels with a gentler approach.

You may also avoid developing diabetes in the first place. About 40 million Americans have a condition called prediabetes, which means your blood sugar is slightly higher than normal. Unless you take steps like exercising, losing weight, and changing your diet, you could develop diabetes. Adopting a low-GI diet can be part of a successful diabetes prevention strategy.

Lose weight the GI way

For people with diabetes, keeping your weight under control is just as important as keeping your blood sugar under control. Obesity and diabetes go hand in hand, with each condition contributing to the other. Fortunately, adopting a low-GI diet can also help you lose weight – whether you have diabetes or not.

Often, high-GI foods, like pastries and other baked goods, are also high in calories. After eating these foods, your blood sugar spikes, then plummets – making you hungry again. Most likely, you reach for another high-GI food to satisfy your hunger, and the cycle continues.

Low-GI foods, like non-starchy vegetables, tend to contain fewer calories, but more nutrients. As an added bonus, foods with low GI values keep you feeling full longer, so you're more satisfied and less likely to overeat. This effect even carries over to your next meal, so making good food choices becomes doubly important.

But even if you eat the same amount of calories, you may lose weight if you swap high-GI foods for low-GI alternatives. Studies show that people who eat low-GI foods, like oatmeal, eggs, low-fat dairy products, produce, and pasta, lose more body fat than those who eat high-GI foods, such as high-fiber cereal products, potatoes, and rice. They also have more success when it comes to keeping off the weight they've lost.

That's probably because the high-GI foods spark an increase in insulin, which moves glucose out of the bloodstream and helps your body convert it to fat for storage. Low-GI foods result in less glucose and less insulin, causing you to burn fat rather than store it.

How often you eat also makes a difference. Two people can eat the same number of calories during the course of a day. But if one person shovels in all those calories in one sitting and the other spreads them out among several small meals and snacks, the effects of those calories will be quite different. Eating smaller, more frequent meals can help improve your blood glucose and cholesterol levels as well as boost your metabolism to help you shed pounds.

Shedding pounds does not mean shedding your favorite foods. Unlike fad diets that severely restrict your food choices, a low glycemic index diet gives you plenty of options — and a better chance for success.

Just remember, you don't have to radically alter your eating habits right away. Make a gradual change to a low-GI diet. Start with small, easy-to-reach goals, like adding more vegetables or fruit. Once you've mastered that, keep tweaking your diet until eating with the glycemic index in mind becomes second nature. You might have a few lapses, but don't get discouraged. Eventually, you'll make a successful transition to a healthy lifelong eating plan.

Of course, any successful weight loss plan must include exercise. While you're revamping your eating habits, make time for more

Sidestep blood sugar spikes

Watch out for high-GI foods that cause your blood sugar to soar — and increase your risk of heart disease. This handy chart helps you avoid foods that are dangerous to people with diabetes. You don't have to eliminate these foods from your diet, but you may want to eat them sparingly.

- bagels
- bread stuffing
- most breakfast cereals
- cheese curls
- cupcake with strawberry icing
- dates
- dinner rolls
- Gatorade sports drink
- Graham crackers
- jellybeans
- Kaiser rolls
- licorice
- Melba toast
- parsnips
- popcorn
- potatoes
- pretzels
- most types of rice
- rice cakes
- scones
- waffles
- watermelon
- white bread

physical activity as well. Exercise speeds up your metabolism so you burn more calories per minute even when you sleep. Exercise also makes your muscles bigger, which makes them better fat-burners. Since you're trying to get rid of extra body fat when you lose weight, combining exercise with a low-GI diet makes a lot of sense. Look for some fun exercise ideas in the chapter *Active Living: Shape up to shake high blood sugar.*

Practical uses for the glycemic index

Now that you understand the glycemic index, you may be wondering how to apply it to everyday life. It may seem complicated at first glance, but just making a few simple changes can have a big effect on your health.

Critics of the GI point out that it's not practical. Rarely do you eat just one food at a time. While researchers have tested some mixed meals, like Lean Cuisine frozen entrées, you have to figure out most food combinations for yourself. You could use a complicated mathematical formula to calculate the GI of your breakfast, lunch, or dinner. But, for most people, that would be more trouble than it's worth. Your best bet is to make smart food choices with the glycemic index as your guide.

Aim for an average daily GI of 50 to 55. But don't get hung up over GI numbers. You don't need to make room for a calculator alongside your knife and fork. As long as you know whether a food is high, medium, or low, that will help. So will these useful strategies.

Switch things up. Swap high GI foods for low GI foods whenever possible. For most high-GI favorites, you can find a tasty low-GI alternative.

▸ If you normally eat potatoes, try sweet potatoes.

▶ Ditch soft white or whole-wheat breads in favor of dense, whole-grain breads. Stone-ground and sourdough breads make good choices.

▶ Instead of crackers, munch on crisp vegetables like carrots, celery, or peppers.

▶ Forget French fries, and opt for a side salad, corn on the cob, or coleslaw instead.

▶ Pass on cakes and pastries and enjoy raisin toast, yogurt, or low-fat mousse for dessert.

▶ Give up hard candy in favor of raisins or other dried fruits. Even chocolate is a better option. Just don't overeat it because it's high in fat.

▶ If you think rice is nice, try basmati or Uncle Ben's converted long-grain rice. Barley, bulgur, quinoa, and pasta make good substitutes, too.

Mix and match. Pair a low GI food with a high GI food to lessen the meal's overall effect on your blood sugar. Some good pairings include:

▶ rice and beans

▶ potatoes and sweet corn

▶ cornflakes and strawberries

Read the fine print. Pay attention to food labels in the supermarket. These helpful boxes can help you make smart decisions.

▶ Don't be fooled by claims like "No added sugar." That doesn't mean the food won't affect your blood sugar.

▶ Note the total carbohydrate, which includes starch, fiber, and sugars. To figure out the available carbohydrate, subtract the fiber from the total carbohydrate.

Find your personal GI

Remember that GI values are averages. Your personal response to a particular food may differ from its published GI. You may want to experiment to see which foods you can handle. When you test your blood sugar, perhaps you will find that potatoes are OK, but peas send your blood sugar through the roof.

▶ Remember to pay attention to calories, fat (especially saturated and trans fats), fiber content, and sodium, too.

Raise the bar. Use your knowledge of the glycemic index to your advantage. In some cases, you may actually want to raise your blood sugar.

▶ Before running a marathon or engaging in another lengthy rigorous exercise, you'll want to eat low GI foods to give your body a steady stream of energy. After your intense workout, you'll want some high GI foods to replenish quickly.

▶ If you are experiencing a bout of hypoglycemia, or low blood sugar, know which foods can give you a quick boost. A half-cup of regular soda or fruit juice, a few jellybeans, or a couple tablespoons of sugar should do the trick. After 15 to 20 minutes, eat a banana or apple or some unsweetened yogurt, or drink a glass of low-fat milk, to keep your blood-sugar levels stable.

Using the glycemic index does not require poring over numbers and formulas. It just involves using your knowledge of relative GI values — low, medium, or high — to enjoy healthy meals.

Choose fun foods to balance blood sugar

If you have diabetes, you need to watch every bit of food that goes in your mouth to keep your blood sugar under control. You may take the same approach if you are trying to lose weight. But that doesn't mean eating can't be fun. When you use the glycemic index to make your food choices, you get a wide range of exciting options. Here's a meal-by-meal look at some tasty low-GI fare.

Breakfast. Skipping breakfast is a common mistake people make when trying to lose weight. The decision to skimp on calories in the morning usually backfires, though, and you end up eating more throughout the day. You need some fuel to jumpstart your day, so start each day with a healthy breakfast.

▶ Eat half a grapefruit or an apple, pear, plum, or orange.

▶ Sip on apple juice, tomato juice, pineapple juice, grapefruit juice, or orange juice.

▶ Enjoy a bowl of a high-fiber, low-GI breakfast cereal, like All-Bran or muesli with low-fat milk. Oatmeal – not the instant kind – is also a good choice.

▶ Top some low-fat yogurt with peaches or strawberries. You can also make a yogurt smoothie with fruit.

▶ Nibble on cottage cheese with orange or grapefruit sections.

▶ Smear some Nutella hazelnut spread or natural peanut butter on whole-grain toast.

Lunch. Keep your energy and blood sugar levels even with a healthy, light lunch. You don't need to give up on sandwiches, as long as you use dense, whole-grain bread and GI-friendly fillings. But you can also branch out and try new things.

▶ Enjoy some soup. Gazpacho, mushroom barley, tomato, lentil, minestrone, and black bean soups will do the trick.

▶ Sink your teeth into a salad. Tabbouleh with tomatoes and cucumber, three-bean salad, Greek salad with feta cheese and olives, or just a big garden salad with lots of vegetables should fill you up. You can also try chicken salad held together with tahini and yogurt, rather than mayonnaise, or a pasta salad with vinaigrette dressing.

▶ Build a sandwich. Start with whole-grain wheat, rye, pumpernickel, or pita bread. Then add peanut butter, turkey or chicken breast, roasted peppers, alfalfa sprouts, hummus, baba ghanoush, or tuna. You could even use lettuce leaves instead of bread to hold your sandwich fillings.

▶ Bite into some fruit. A peach, pear, or plum provides a perfect ending to a mid-day meal.

Dinner. Your last meal of the day does not have to be the biggest. But it should include mostly vegetables, plus at least one low-GI carbohydrate, along with your protein.

▶ Go green. Enjoy a mixed green salad or a Caprese salad of tomato, mozzarella, and basil. You can also try arugula, watercress, or bean salads.

▶ Get your protein from lean meats, fish, and poultry. Try grilled fish in lemon butter sauce or roast pork loin. You can also eat beans, peas, or lentils for your protein.

▶ Try tasty dishes like pasta with white clam sauce, barley seafood risotto, or a tofu vegetable stir-fry.

▶ Save room for dessert. Mix fruits with low-fat versions of pudding, ice cream, or yogurt to end your meal in style.

Snacks. If you eat several small meals each day instead of three big ones, you'll need an occasional snack to adjust your blood sugar levels.

▶ Put peanut butter on a celery stalk, or dip raw vegetables in a dip like hummus, baba ghanoush, or guacamole.

▶ Grab a handful of homemade trail mix of nuts, seeds, and dried fruits. Plain nuts and olives also make good snacks.

▶ Enjoy pickled or hard-boiled eggs.

▶ Munch on fresh fruit, either whole or sliced. Apples, grapes, oranges, pears, and plums really hit the spot.

▶ Indulge in a small square of dark chocolate. Chocolate is actually a low-GI food – you just don't want to eat too much of it because of its high fat content.

Think of eating as an adventure and a challenge. Each meal – and mid-meal snack – gives you an opportunity to experiment with healthy, yummy foods while keeping your blood sugar levels and weight under control. Bon appetit.

Smart tips for restaurant eating

With a handy glycemic index chart, you can shop for low-GI foods in the supermarket and cook low-GI meals at home. But even when you dine out or have to eat on the go, you don't have to abandon your low-GI diet. It just takes some resourcefulness. Follow these tips for enjoying healthy meals away from home.

▶ Pass on the pre-meal basket of bread. If you want an appetizer, choose one with vegetables or meat instead. You could also have a cup of soup.

▶ Order a salad as your entrée, but hold the bread and croutons. Lean meats, fish, and poultry also make good main courses.

▶ Choose sautéed or steamed vegetables as your sides.

▶ Share an entrée with a friend so you don't pig out on a mammoth portion of food.

▸ Have only a small taste of dessert. Share the rest with your dining companions, or take it home to eat gradually over the course of the week.

▸ Play it smart at fast food restaurants. Go for the salads — but watch out for high-GI extras like crunchy noodles — or get a burger and ditch the bun. Opt for water instead of a sugary drink, and never super-size anything.

▸ Be careful at buffets. Skip the breads, cereals, and pastries, and focus on offerings like salads, vegetables, prime rib, and salmon. Eat slowly and only refill your plate with tiny morsels if you're still hungry.

▸ Branch out. Ethnic restaurants often have good low-GI choices. Try sushi, a tortilla with beans and tomato sauce, Thai noodles

Expand options with ethnic foods

Broaden your horizons, and you'll broaden your food choices. Ethnic restaurants represent some of your best options for healthy restaurant dining. Japanese, Thai, and Indian cuisines feature mainly low-GI choices. Just beware of canned lychees, fried foods, and heavy, buttery sauces.

Chinese restaurants have several vegetable dishes on the menu. You do have to limit the sticky white rice, though. That can send your blood sugar through the roof.

In Mexican and Italian restaurants, order wisely and limit the chips or bread. Grilled seafood or chicken dishes, black beans, and fajitas make good Mexican choices. Pasta, seafood, and meat dishes can be healthy as long as they are not smothered in cheese. So can thin-crust pizza with vegetable toppings.

with vegetables, lentil soup, stuffed grape leaves, tabbouleh, hummus, or Moroccan couscous with chickpeas.

▶ Speak up. If you can't find any low-GI choices on the menu, you can always ask your server for something you can eat. Most places will be happy to oblige you. After all, the customer is always right.

▶ Pack a low-GI lunch. Make sandwiches on dense, whole-grain bread — or try an open-face sandwich with one slice of bread instead of two.

▶ Snack sensibly. Carry low-GI snacks like nuts, dried apricots, raisins, an orange or apple, grapes, beef jerky, raw carrots, celery, or radishes, olives, and hard cheeses.

Whether you're on the road for business or looking for a pleasurable night on the town, you should be able to find a tasty, low-GI meal.

Savvy cooking saves old favorites

Keep the glycemic index in mind when you're shopping at the supermarket or ordering a meal in a restaurant. But some of the most important GI strategies take place right in your own kitchen. For example, you can change how starchy foods like rice and potatoes affect blood sugar levels just by changing the way you cook them.

▶ Chill out. Serve potatoes cold. Boiled and cooled potatoes have a gentler effect on you blood sugar and insulin response than hot, freshly boiled potatoes. That's because chilling the cooked potatoes increases their resistant starch, the kind that resists digestion.

▶ Add some acid. Splash a vinegar dressing on your cooled potatoes to lower their GI even more. The vinegar's acidity helps slow digestion. Citrus juices, like lemon juice, do the same thing. For variety and flavor, try apple cider, balsamic, red wine, or herb-infused vinegars with your cooked veggies, pasta sauces,

Search Web sites for more info

For more information on the glycemic index, including a search-able index of foods, check out *www.glycemicindex.com*, a Web site maintained by the University of Sydney.

Freelance medical writer and diabetes specialist David Mendosa also has an informative Web page devoted to the glycemic index at *www.mendosa.com/gi.htm*.

dips, and grilled meats. Just 4 teaspoons of vinegar can lower blood sugar by 30 percent.

▶ Increase the pressure. According to a Danish study, pressure par-boiled rice lowered the GI by nearly 30 percent compared to non-parboiled rice.

▶ Know when to say when. Do not overcook pasta. Pasta cooked al dente, or firm to the teeth, has a lower GI. It also tastes better than mushy macaroni.

▶ Boil it down. A Jamaican study found that foods roasted or baked had higher GI values than those boiled or fried. The study included various yams, potatoes, and plantains.

You don't have to say goodbye to old favorites like pasta, potatoes, and rice. With a few simple cooking adjustments, you can make these starchy foods more GI-friendly.

GI: an important piece of your dietary puzzle

Think of your diet as a jigsaw puzzle. As helpful as the glycemic index is, remember it is only one aspect of a healthy diet, or one piece of that puzzle.

If you use only the glycemic index when choosing your food, it does not always make sense. In other words, not all high-GI foods are bad and not all low-GI foods are good. Some high-GI foods, like bread and potatoes, provide nutrition and can be part of a healthy diet. Conversely, a low-GI food could be high in saturated fat, like sausage, or devoid of any nutritional value, like diet soda.

To complete your dietary puzzle, you need to pay attention to total calories, the type of fat you're eating, the sodium and fiber content of your food, and the important nutrients your food provides.

Still, the glycemic index represents a useful guide for people with diabetes or at risk of developing diabetes, people who want to lose weight, and people who just want to eat healthy. It may be just one piece of the puzzle – but it's a very important piece.

Use the following tables compiled from the Sydney University Glycemic Index Research Service (SUGiRS) and several manufacturers to find the glycemic index and load of your favorite foods. If you can't find a GI value for a food you eat often, you may want to contact the manufacturer and ask them to have the GI tested by an accredited laboratory such as SUGiRS. You will find current information and updates on the university's GI Web site at *www.glycemicindex.com.*

Food	GI Rating	GI (Glucose=100)	Approx. serving size	Available carbs (g) per serving	GL rating	GL
Bakery products						
Apple muffin	Low	44	60g	29	Medium	13
Banana cake	Low	47	80g	38	Medium	18
Chocolate cake, with frosting	Low	38	111g	52	High	20
Pound cake	Low	54	53g	28	Medium	15
Sponge cake	Low	46	63g	36	Medium	17
Vanilla cake, with frosting	Low	42	111g	58	High	24
Angel food cake	Medium	67	50g	29	Medium	19
Blueberry muffin	Medium	59	57g	29	Medium	17
Bran muffin	Medium	60	57g	24	Medium	15
Carrot muffin	Medium	62	57g	32	High	20
Pastry pie crust	Medium	59	57g	26	Medium	15
Corn muffin, low-amylose	High	102	57g	29	High	30
Doughnut	High	76	47g	23	Medium	17
Scones	High	92	25g	9	Low	7
Beverages						
Apple juice, unsweetened	Low	40	8 oz	29	Medium	12
Grapefruit juice, unsweetened	Low	48	8 oz	20	Low	9
Orange juice, unsweetened	Low	50	8 oz	26	Medium	13
Orange sports drink, Allsport	Low	53	8 oz	17	Low	9
Pineapple juice, unsweetened	Low	46	8 oz	34	Medium	16
Smoothie, raspberry	Low	33	8 oz	41	Medium	14
Tomato juice, canned	Low	38	8 oz	9	Low	4
Coca-cola	Medium	63	8 oz	26	Medium	16
Cranberry juice cocktail	Medium	68	8 oz	35	High	24
Orange juice, reconstituted	Medium	57	8 oz	26	Medium	15
Fruit punch	High	95	12 oz	44	High	42
Breads						
Buckwheat bread	Low	47	30 g	21	Low	10

Food	GI Rating	GI (Glucose=100)	Approx. serving size	Available carbs (g) per serving	GL rating	GL
Breads						
Cracked wheat bulgur bread	Low	53	30 g	20	Medium	11
Healthy Choice Hearty 7 Grain bread	Low	55	30 g	14	Low	8
Muesli bread, made from package	Low	54	30 g	12	Low	7
Pumpernickel bread	Low	46	30 g	11	Low	5
Sourdough rye bread	Low	53	30 g	12	Low	6
Soy and linseed bread, made from package	Low	50	30 g	10	Low	5
Barley flour bread (100%)	Medium	67	30 g	13	Low	9
Croissant	Medium	67	57 g	25	Medium	17
Hamburger bun	Medium	61	30 g	15	Low	9
Healthy Choice Hearty 100% Whole Grain bread	Medium	62	30 g	14	Low	9
Hunger Filler bread, Natural Ovens	Medium	59	30 g	13	Low	7
Light rye bread	Medium	68	30 g	14	Low	10
Nutty Natural Whole Grain bread, Natural Ovens	Medium	59	30 g	12	Low	7
Oat bread, coarse	Medium	65	30 g	19	Medium	12
Pita bread, white	Medium	57	30 g	17	Low	10
Taco shell, Old El Paso	Medium	68	20 g	12	Low	8
White bread, high fiber	Medium	68	30 g	13	Low	9
Whole meal rye bread	Medium	58	30 g	14	Low	8
Bagel	High	72	70 g	35	High	25
Bread stuffing	High	74	30 g	21	Medium	16

Food	GI Rating	GI (Glucose=100)	Approx. serving size	Available carbs (g) per serving	GL rating	GL
Breads						
English muffin bread, Natural Ovens	High	77	30 g	14	Medium	11
French baguette	High	95	30 g	15	Medium	15
Gluten-free white bread, sliced	High	80	30 g	15	Medium	12
Kaiser roll	High	73	30 g	16	Medium	12
White bread	High	70	30 g	14	Low	10
White bread, whole-meal flour	High	73	30 g	14	Low	10
White bread, Wonder	High	73	30 g	14	Low	10
Breakfast cereals and related products						
All-Bran, Kellogg's	Low	38	30 g	23	Low	9
Bran Buds, with psyllium, Kellogg's	Low	47	30 g	12	Low	6
Frosties, cornflakes, Kellogg's	Low	55	30 g	26	Medium	15
Muesli, toasted, Purina	Low	43	30 g	17	Low	7
Bran Chex, Nabisco	Medium	58	30 g	19	Medium	11
Cream of Wheat, Nabisco	Medium	66	250 g	26	Medium	17
Fruit Loops, Kellogg's	Medium	69	30 g	26	Medium	18
Life, Quaker Oats	Medium	66	30 g	25	Medium	15
Oatmeal, mix, Quaker Oats	Medium	69	50 g	35	High	24
Oatmeal, 1 minute, Quaker Oats	Medium	66	250 g	26	Medium	17
Puffed wheat, Quaker Oats	Medium	67	30 g	20	Medium	13
Raisin Bran, Kellogg's	Medium	61	30 g	19	Medium	12
Special K, Kellogg's	Medium	69	30 g	21	Medium	14
Bran Flakes, Kellogg's	High	74	30 g	18	Medium	13
Cheerios, General Mills	High	74	30 g	20	Medium	15

Food	GI Rating	GI (Glucose=100)	Approx. serving size	Available carbs (g) per serving	GL rating	GL
Breakfast cereals and related products						
Coco Pops, Kellogg's	High	77	30 g	26	High	20
Corn Bran, Kellogg's	High	75	30 g	20	Medium	15
Corn Chex, Nabisco	High	83	30 g	25	High	21
Corn Flakes, Kellogg's	High	92	30 g	26	High	24
Cream of Wheat, instant, Nabisco	High	74	250 g	30	High	22
Crispix, Kellogg's	High	87	30 g	25	High	22
Golden Grahams, General Mills	High	71	30 g	25	Medium	18
Grapenuts Flakes, Post	High	80	30 g	22	Medium	17
Grapenuts, Post	High	71	30 g	22	Medium	16
Oatmeal, rolled oats	High	75	250 g	23	Medium	17
Pop Tarts, double chocolate, Kellogg's	High	70	50 g	35	High	24
Rice Chex, Nabisco	High	89	30 g	26	High	23
Rice Krispies, Kellogg's	High	82	30 g	26	High	22
Shredded Wheat, Nabisco	High	75	30 g	20	Medium	15
Total, General Mills	High	76	30 g	22	Medium	17
Waffles, Aunt Jemima	High	76	35 g	13	Low	10
Wheatabix	High	75	30 g	22	Medium	16
Cereal grains						
Barley, pearled	Low	25	150 g	42	Medium	11
Buckwheat	Low	54	150 g	30	Medium	16
Corn, sweet, frozen, reheated	Low	47	150 g	33	Medium	16
Corn, sweet, whole kernel, canned	Low	46	150 g	28	Low	1.3
Quinoa, organic, boiled	Low	53	100 g	17	Low	9

Food	GI Rating	GI (Glucose=100)	Approx. serving size	Available carbs (g) per serving	GL rating	GL
Cereal grains						
Rice, brown	Low	55	150 g	33	Medium	18
Rice, Cajun Style, Uncle Ben's	Low	51	150 g	37	Medium	19
Rice, white, converted long grain	Low	47	150 g	36	Medium	17
Corn, sweet	Medium	60	150 g	33	High	20
Cornmeal	Medium	69	150 g	13	Low	9
Couscous	Medium	65	150 g	35	High	23
Rice, basmati, boiled, Mahatma	Medium	58	150 g	38	High	22
Rice, long grain	Medium	56	150 g	41	High	23
Rice, white	Medium	64	150 g	36	High	23
Rice, white, instant	Medium	69	150 g	42	High	29
Cookies						
FIFTY 50 Butter	Low	36	NA	20	Low	7.2
FIFTY 50 Chocolate Chip	Low	34	NA	17	Low	5.8
FIFTY 50 Fudge Brownie	Low	33	NA	23	Low	7.6
FIFTY 50 Oatmeal	Low	30	NA	20	Low	6
FIFTY 50 Vanilla Creme Filled Wafers	Low	41	NA	27	Medium	11.1
Oatmeal	Low	54	25 g	17	Low	9
Peanut Butter, FIFTY 50	Low	32	NA	19	Low	6.1
Arrowroot, McCormick's	Medium	65	NA	19	Medium	12
Shortbread	Medium	64	NA	16	Low	10
Vanilla wafers	High	77	NA	18	Medium	14
Crackers						
Cheddar Cheese Crackers, Combos Snacks	Low	54	48 g	30.5	Medium	16.5
Breton Wheat Crackers	Medium	67	25 g	14	Low	10

Food	GI Rating	GI (Glucose=100)	Approx. serving size	Available carbs (g) per serving	GL rating	GL
Crackers						
Rye crispbread	Medium	63	25 g	16	Low	10
Ryvita	Medium	69	25 g	16	Medium	11
Stoned Wheat Thins	Medium	67	25 g	17	Medium	12
Water Cracker	Medium	63	25 g	18	Medium	11
Kavli Norwegian Crispbread	High	71	25 g	16	Medium	12
Melba Toast	High	70	30 g	23	Medium	16
Premium Soda Cracker	High	74	25 g	17	Medium	12
Rice Cakes	High	78	3 pcs	21	Medium	17
Rice Crackers	High	91	25 g	19.9	Medium	18
Dairy products and alternatives						
Custard	Low	38	100 g	16	Low	6
Ice cream, lowfat, vanilla	Low	50	50 g	6	Low	3
Ice cream, premium, chocolate	Low	37	50 g	9	Low	4
Milk, chocolate, lowfat	Low	34	250 mL	26	Low	9
Milk, full-fat	Low	27	250 g	12	Low	3
Milk, lowfat, chocolate	Low	24	250 g	15	Low	3
Milk, skim	Low	32	250 g	13	Low	4
Milk, soy, 1.5 - 3.0% fat	Low	44	250 mL	17	Low	8
Mousse, reduced fat	Low	34	50 g	10	Low	4
Pudding, instant	Low	44	100 g	16	Low	7
Soy yogurt, 2% fat, fruit	Low	50	200 g	26	Medium	13
Yogurt, lowfat, black cherry	Low	41	150 g	21.5	Low	9
Yogurt, lowfat, aspartame	Low	14	200 g	13	Low	2
Yogurt, sweetened, fruit	Low	33	200 mL	31	Low	10
Yogurt, vanilla, reduced-fat	Low	26	200 g	10	Low	3
Figs, dried	Medium	61	60 g	26	Medium	16
Ice cream, regular	Medium	61	50 g	13	Low	8

Food	GI Rating	GI (Glucose=100)	Approx. serving size	Available carbs (g) per serving	GL rating	GL
Dairy products and alternatives						
Milk, condensed, sweetened	Medium	61	250 g	136	High	83
Dates, dried	High	103	60 g	40	High	42
Fruits and fruit products						
Apple	Low	40	120 g	16	Low	6
Apple, dried	Low	29	60 g	34	Low	10
Apricots, dried	Low	32	60 g	30	Low	10
Banana, overripe	Low	48	120 g	25	Medium	12
Banana, ripe	Low	51	120 g	25	Medium	13
Banana, slightly underripe	Low	42	120 g	25	Medium	11
Cherries, fresh	Low	22	120 g	12	Low	3
Fruit cocktail, canned	Low	55	120 g	16	Low	9
Grapefruit, fresh	Low	25	120 g	11	Low	3
Grapes	Low	43	120 g	17	Low	7
Jam, strawberry	Low	51	30 g	20	Low	10
Kiwifruit, fresh	Low	53	120 g	12	Low	6
Mango, fresh	Low	51	120 g	15	Low	8
Marmalade, orange	Low	48	30 g	20	Low	9
Oranges, fresh	Low	48	120 g	11	Low	5
Peach, canned in juice	Low	38	120 g	11	Low	4
Peach, canned in light syrup	Low	52	120 g	18	Low	9
Peach, fresh	Low	42	120 g	11	Low	5
Pear, canned in pear juice	Low	44	120 g	11	Low	5
Pear, fresh	Low	41	120 g	8	Low	3
Plum, fresh	Low	39	120 g	12	Low	5
Prunes, pitted	Low	29	60 g	33	Low	10
Strawberries, fresh	Low	40	120 g	3	Low	1
Apricots, canned in light syrup	Medium	64	120 g	19	Medium	12

Food	GI Rating	GI (Glucose=100)	Approx. serving size	Available carbs (g) per serving	GL rating	GL
Fruit and fruit products						
Apricots, fresh	Medium	57	120 g	9	Low	5
Breadfruit	Medium	68	120 g	27	Medium	18
Cantaloupe, fresh	Medium	65	120 g	6	Low	4
Papaya, fresh	Medium	59	120 g	17	Low	10
Pineapple. fresh	Medium	59	120 g	13	Low	7
Raisins	Medium	64	60 g	44	High	28
Sultanas	Medium	56	60 g	45	High	25
Watermelon, fresh	High	72	120 g	6	Low	4
Legumes and nuts						
Baked beans	Low	48	150 g	15	Low	7
Black beans, cooked 45 min.	Low	20	150 g	25	Low	5
Black-eyed peas, boiled	Low	42	150 g	30	Medium	13
Butter beans, cooked	Low	36	150 g	20	Low	6
Chickpeas, boiled	Low	28	150 g	30	Low	8
Chickpeas, canned in brine	Low	42	150 g	22	Low	9
Haricot and navy beans	Low	39	150 g	30	Medium	12
Kidney beans	Low	23	150 g	25	Low	6
Lentils	Low	29	150 g	18	Low	5
Lentils, green, boiled	Low	22	150 g	18	Low	4
Lima beans, baby, frozen, reheated	Low	32	150 g	30	Low	10
Mung beans, boiled 20 min.	Low	31	150 g	17	Low	5
Pinto beans, boiled	Low	39	150 g	26	Low	10
Soya beans, boiled	Low	18	150 g	6	Low	1
Split pea, yellow, boiled	Low	32	150 g	19	Low	6
Mixed meals and convenience foods						
Chicken nuggets, frozen, reheated	Low	46	100 g	16	Low	7

Food	GI Rating	GI (Glucose=100)	Approx. serving size	Available carbs (g) per serving	GL rating	GL
Mixed meals and convenience foods						
Fish sticks	Low	38	100 g	19	Low	7
Pizza, Super Supreme, Thin and Crispy, Pizza Hut	Low	30	100 g	22	Low	7
Spaghetti bolognaise	Low	52	360 g	48	High	25
Sushi, sea algae, vinegar, rice	Low	55	100 g	37	High	20
Sushi, salmon	Low	48	100 g	36	Medium	17
Pizza	Medium	60	100 g	27	Medium	16
Stir-fried vegetables with chicken and boiled white rice	High	73	360 g	75	High	55
Nutritional-support products						
Choice, vanilla	Low	23	237 mL	24	Low	6
Ensure	Low	50	237 mL	40	Medium	19
Ensure bar, chocolate fudge brownie	Low	48	38 g	20	Low	8
Ensure pudding, vanilla	Low	36	113 g	26	Low	9
Glucerna, vanilla	Low	31	237 mL	23	Low	7
Ultracal with fiber	Low	40	237 mL	29	Medium	12
Enercal Plus, powder	Medium	61	237 mL	40	Medium	19
Pasta and noodles						
Capellini	Low	45	180 g	45	High	20
Cheese tortellini	Low	50	180 g	21	Low	10
Fettuccine, egg	Low	40	180 g	46	Medium	18
Fusilli, boiled for 10 min.	Low	54	50 g	36.3	High	20
Gluten-free pasta, boiled 8 min.	Low	54	180 g	42	High	22
Instant noodles	Low	47	180 g	40	Medium	19
Lasagne, boiled 10 min.	Low	55	50 g	36	High	20
Linguine, thick, wheat flour	Low	46	180 g	48	High	22

Food	GI Rating	GI (Glucose=100)	Approx. serving size	Available carbs (g) per serving	GL rating	GL
Pasta and noodles						
Linguine, thin, wheat flour	Low	52	180 g	45	High	23
Macaroni, plain, boiled 5 min.	Low	45	180 g	49	High	22
Meat ravioli	Low	39	180 g	38	Medium	15
Mung bean noodles	Low	39	180 g	45	Medium	18
Rice noodles, fresh, boiled	Low	40	180 g	39	Medium	15
Spaghetti, boiled 10-15 min.	Low	44	180 g	48	High	21
Spaghetti, boiled 5 min.	Low	38	180 g	48	Medium	18
Spirali, wheat, boiled to al dente	Low	43	180 g	44	Medium	19
Vermicelli, white, boiled	Low	35	180 g	44	Medium	16
Gnocchi	Medium	68	180 g	48	High	33
Macaroni and cheese (packaged)	Medium	64	180 g	51	High	32
Spaghetti, boiled 20 min.	Medium	61	180 g	44	High	27
Snack foods and confectionery						
Cashew nuts, salted	Low	22	50 g	13	Low	3
Chocolate and Vanilla Carb Smart Ice Cream, Nestle	Low	32	48 g	2.2	Low	0.7
Ice cream, premium, French vanilla	Low	38	50 g	9	Low	3
M & M Peanut Candies	Low	33	30 g	17	Low	6
Milk Chocolate Bar, FIFTY 50	Low	30	NA	21	Low	6.3
Nutella	Low	33	20 g	12	Low	4
Peanuts	Low	14	50 g	6	Low	1
Snack bar, apple cinnamon	Low	40	50 g	29	Medium	12
Snack bar, peanut butter and chocolate chip	Low	37	50 g	27	Low	10

Food	GI Rating	GI (Glucose=100)	Approx. serving size	Available carbs (g) per serving	GL rating	GL
Snack foods and confectionery						
Snickers bar	Low	55	60 g	35	Medium	19
Twix Cookie Bar	Low	44	60 g	39	Medium	17
Vanilla Carb Smart Ice Cream, Nestle	Low	7	48 g	2.3	Low	0.2
Corn chips	Medium	63	50 g	26	Medium	17
Mars candy bar	Medium	65	60 g	40	High	26
Potato chips	Medium	57	50 g	18	Low	10
Whole grain chocolate chip bars, Kudos	Medium	62	50 g	32	High	20
Fruit roll-ups	High	99	30 g	25	High	24
Jelly beans	High	78	30 g	28	High	22
Peppermint candy, Lifesavers	High	70	30 g	30	High	21
Popcorn, plain, microwaved	High	72	20 g	11	Low	8
Pretzels, wheat, oven-baked	High	83	30 g	20	Medium	16
Skittles	High	70	50 g	45	High	32
Sugar, granulated	High	84	1 tsp	4	High	34
Soups						
Lentil soup	Low	44	250 mL	21	Low	9
Minestrone soup	Low	39	250 mL	187	Low	7
Tomato soup	Low	38	250 mL	17	Low	6
Black bean soup	Medium	64	250 mL	27	Medium	17
Green pea soup	Medium	66	250 mL	41	High	27
Split pea soup	Medium	60	250 mL	27	Medium	16
Sports bars						
Ironman PR Bar, chocolate	Low	39	65 g	26	Low	10
Power Bar	Medium	56	65 g	42	High	24
Sugars and sugar alcohols						
Fructose	Low	19	10 g	10	Low	2

Food	GI Rating	GI (Glucose=100)	Approx. serving size	Available carbs (g) per serving	GL rating	GL
Sugars and sugar alcohols						
Honey	Low	55	28 g	18	Low	10
Lactose	Low	46	10 g	10	Low	5
Low Cal Fruit Spread, FIFTY 50	Low	6	NA	4	Low	0.24
Maple Syrup, FIFTY 50	Low	19	NA	18	Low	3.42
Xylitol	Low	8	10 g	10	Low	1
Sucrose	Medium	68	10 g	10	Low	7
Glucose	High	99	10 g	10	Low	10
Maltose	High	105	10 g	10	Medium	11
Vegetables (including roots and tubers)						
Carrots, boiled	Low	47	80 g	6	Low	3
Green peas	Low	48	80 g	7	Low	3
Potato, white, boiled or cooked	Low	50	150 g	28	Medium	14
Sweet corn	Low	54	80 g	17	Low	9
Taro, boiled	Low	55	150 g	8	Low	4
Yam, boiled	Low	37	150 g	36	Medium	13
Beetroot	Medium	64	80 g	7	Low	5
New potato	Medium	57	150 g	21	Medium	12
Sweet potato	Medium	61	150 g	28	Medium	17
Broad beans	High	79	80 g	11	Low	9
French fries, frozen, reheated	High	75	150 g	29	High	22
Parsnips	High	97	80 g	12	Medium	12
Potato, instant mashed	High	85	150 g	20	Medium	17
Potato, mashed	High	74	150 g	20	Medium	15
Potato, Russet, baked	High	85	150 g	30	High	26
Pumpkin	High	75	80 g	4	Low	3
Rutabaga	High	72	150 g	10	Low	7
Tapioca, boiled with milk	High	81	250 g	18	Medium	14

Diet Defense

Smart eating to balance blood sugar

Smart eating strategies

It may seem like diabetes is all about what you can't eat. In fact, fighting it has just as much to do with what you should eat as what you shouldn't.

Food and nutrients actually help your body regulate blood sugar and make the most of insulin. Certain compounds in food can even work like insulin in your body. What you eat can improve your insulin sensitivity, balance blood sugar spikes, and help prevent as well as treat diabetes.

Sometimes battling this disease is a matter of making smart food choices, like munching almonds instead of potato chips, or making pancakes with buckwheat flour instead of white flour. Other times, it's about adding specific foods to your diet, such as cherries. Whether you are worried about developing diabetes or need help managing it now, there's a food to help you.

This eating advice will help you maintain a healthy weight, control your blood sugar, and avoid dangerous complications.

▶ Eat more healthy carbohydrates, like sweet fruits, crunchy vegetables, legumes, low-fat milk, and whole grains.

▶ Limit saturated fats to less than 7 percent of your total calories. You'll find them in meat, egg yolks, whole milk, butter, cream, and cheese.

▶ Avoid trans fats. Check package labels to find where trans fats lurk.

▶ Cut cholesterol to less than 200 milligrams a day.

▶ Eat fish at least twice a week. Make it baked, broiled, or blackened, but not fried.

▶ Be sure you understand serving sizes. Weigh and measure your food if you need to.

▶ Eat roughly the same amount of food at the same time each day to keep your blood sugar steady. Stick to a schedule for meals and snacks, and do not skip meals.

You won't find a magic, one-size-fits-all diabetes diet, but you can discover the best plan for you by working with a registered dietitian or certified diabetes educator. Your goal is to keep your blood sugar from getting too high or too low. Ask your doctor how many meals and snacks you should eat and how often to check your blood sugar. And make sure you discuss any big changes in the way you eat with him first.

Top foods that fight diabetes

Some foods may cause type 2 diabetes if you eat too much of them. Eating lots of foods with a high glycemic index, like white bread, crackers, and cake, raises your risk. So does a diet heavy on meat, especially red meat and fatty foods.

Other foods help prevent diabetes and its complications as well as manage the disease if you already have it. Throughout this chapter, you'll learn more information on these healing staples for diabetes. In the meantime, start stocking your cabinets so you always have these foods in your pantry.

▶ apples

▶ apricots

▶ artichokes

▶ avocados

▶ black beans

▶ blueberries

▶ bran flakes cereal

▶ broccoli

▶ green tea

▶ chili pepper

▶ guava jelly

▶ lentils

▶ low-fat milk

▶ oatmeal

▶ olive oil

▶ oranges

- brown rice
- buckwheat flour
- bulgur
- cherries
- cinnamon
- coffee
- cornstarch
- curry powder
- dark chocolate
- fenugreek
- flaxseeds
- garlic
- peanut butter
- psyllium seeds
- rainbow trout
- Red Bush tea
- salmon
- skinless poultry
- strawberries
- sweet potatoes
- sweet red peppers
- tomato juice
- vinegar
- walnuts

Fill up on fiber to fight diabetes

Your grandparents may have called it roughage, but fiber actually helps your body run more smoothly. This vital staple helps slow down the rate at which starch and sugar are absorbed into the bloodstream. And wait until you hear what it does for your weight.

Pioneering British surgeon Denis Burkitt uncovered this amazing health secret while working in Africa during the 1940s. He noticed that several diseases common in industrialized countries were rare in rural Africa – constipation, gallstones, hemorrhoids, diverticulosis, varicose veins, appendicitis, and hiatal hernias.

The difference, he explained, was diet. People in developing nations tended to eat about 60 grams of fiber a day compared to the 20 grams or less eaten in Western countries. He realized that "dietary fiber," a term he coined, has remarkable properties that help the body avoid disease.

Fiber comes in two main varieties – soluble and insoluble. Soluble fiber, which dissolves in water, can be found in dried beans and peas, oats, barley, flaxseed, and many fruits and vegetables. You can find insoluble fiber, which does not dissolve in water, in whole-grain breads and cereals as well as fruits and veggies with rough, chewy textures.

Your body can't break down insoluble fiber, but it does become mushy and moves without delay through your digestive system, keeping your bowels working smoothly and toning your digestive muscles. Many foods contain both soluble fiber and insoluble fiber, and both kinds offer many health benefits, including these.

Defends against diabetes. Fiber helps your body absorb sugars and starches more slowly. This means your blood sugar rises gradually over a longer period, instead of skyrocketing after a meal. As a result, fiber keeps a cap on sugar spikes.

Fights weight gain. Like a sponge, fiber absorbs water and swells, making you feel full long after you eat it. As a result, you may eat less and skip fattening snacks and desserts. But that's not all. According to Burkitt, the more bulky, high-fiber foods you eat, the less fat you'll consume.

Protects against heart attack and stroke. Soluble fiber in foods like carrots, lentils, oatmeal, and oat bran helps eliminate much of the artery-clogging cholesterol that can cause a heart attack or stroke. How? This type of fiber turns soft in your body, slowing things down in your stomach and small intestine. Soluble fiber sweeps cholesterol up and whisks it away, which helps lower the cholesterol levels in your blood. A study of 21,000 men in Finland found that those who ate an average of 35 grams of fiber a day had 25 percent fewer heart attacks than men who averaged just 16 grams a day.

Types of fiber		
	Insoluble	**Soluble**
Characteristics	Does not dissolve	Dissolves in water
Action	Adds bulk; speeds up trip through your digestive system	Makes food soft and gummy so it moves through your system easier
Best sources	Whole wheat breads & cereals, brown rice, beans, popcorn, celery, corn	Oats, barley, peas, beans, certain fruits, pectin, psyllium

Lowers high blood pressure. Some researchers think taking in 12 grams of soluble fiber every day might help lower high blood pressure. To get these amazing benefits, stick with this sure-fire fiber advice.

▸ Increase your fiber intake gradually. Too much, too quickly can lead to bloating, gas, diarrhea, and cramps. It's also important to drink plenty of water with a high-fiber diet.

▸ Try to get 30 grams of fiber a day for men and 21 grams for women, after age 49. You can go as high as 35 grams before it begins to interfere with your ability to absorb iron, calcium, zinc, and copper. However, most Americans get only 5 to 20 grams of fiber daily.

▸ Aim for a good mix of soluble and insoluble fiber. Both types provide a variety of health benefits.

▸ Think food first. Foods are better for you and tastier than fiber supplements, which don't contain vital nutrients and can deplete your body of iron and calcium.

▸ Discover the "wrapping." Whenever possible, wash fruits and veggies and eat the skin, as well as the tasty insides.

Go fish for whole-body health

It's not just a leisurely pastime or even a card game. Fishing is now first aid. Whether you hook them at the lake or at the super-market, using God's gift from the sea can help prevent over 15 ailments, including arthritis, heart disease, cancer, and type 2 diabetes. Best of all, you can get this remedy in any grocery store.

Eating fish at least three times a week can slash your risk of diabetes and heart problems. And thanks to healthy fats that prevent blood clots and improve your circulation, you could cut your stroke risk in half. In fact, the American Heart Association prescribes fish as a first line of treatment for warding off high blood pressure and heart attacks. Baked or broiled, fish is a nutritional winner. It's low in artery-clogging saturated fats, cholesterol, and calories, and loaded with amazing unsaturated fats, vitamins, and minerals.

Reap the benefits of omega-3. Some types of fat such as trans and saturated fats can be hard on your heart and raise your cholesterol. But others known as unsaturated fats actually seem to control your cholesterol and keep your heart young and strong. Omega-3 fatty acids are a kind of polyunsaturated fat (PUFA) in fish that give your arteries a much-needed break, and some experts believe a fish-filled diet could keep your mind sharp as you age. That means a fishy diet could kill two diseases with one stone, lowering your risk of heart disease and Alzheimer's.

Just one serving of fatty fish a week can significantly reduce your heart attack risk – even for diabetics and smokers. A large study on male doctors found that those who ate at least one fish meal a week were 52 percent less likely to die from a sudden heart attack than those who ate fish less than once a month.

Experts with the American Heart Association say the omega-3 in fish can have a huge impact on your heart. Eaten regularly, these super fats:

▶ rein in high blood pressure.

▶ reduce triglyceride levels.

▶ lower your chances for dangerous blood clots.

▶ slow down plaque build-up in your arteries.

▶ decrease your risk of arrhythmia – irregular heartbeat – and of sudden heart-related death.

The protective effects of fishy omega-3 fatty acids kick in quickly. Even if you haven't eaten fish all your life, you could start now and still reap the benefits just by serving up fatty fish twice a week. It's amazing but true. Just two servings a week can fight depression, heart attack, stroke, diabetes, and cancer. (Hint: one serving means a cooked filet about the size of a deck of cards.) People who already have heart disease should talk to their doctor about healthy diet changes – like adding more fish to help get their illness under control.

Reel in Atlantic salmon, herring, mackerel, sardines, or rainbow trout for the most omega-3 fatty acids. The firm, darker species of fish often have more omega-3 fats than fish with white flesh. Remove the skin before cooking it. This won't affect the omega-3 content, but it will lower the overall fat content. You can further up your intake by broiling or baking your fish with omega-3-rich canola or soybean oil, and adding English walnuts or ground flaxseed to your meals. Remember, fried fish doesn't count.

Iron out the kinks. It's often associated with strength, and no wonder. Iron is your body's packhorse, carrying life-giving oxygen with your blood to your muscles and other body parts. If you're low on this mineral, you'll notice. You'll feel too tired to climb out of bed and too weak to face the day.

Best fish sources for more omega-3

For your best sources of omega-3, check this chart. Portions are based on an uncooked serving size of 100 grams — approximately 3 to 3 1/2 ounces.

Food	Omega-3 in grams	% omega-3 in total fat	Total fat in grams
Sardines in oil	3.3	21	15.5
Pacific herring	1.7	12	13.9
Atlantic herring	1.6	18	9.0
Lake trout	1.6	17	9.7
European anchovy	1.4	29	4.8
Atlantic salmon	1.2	22	5.4
Pink salmon	1.0	29	3.4
Striped bass	0.8	35	2.3
Pacific oyster	0.6	26	2.3
Blue mussels	0.5	22	2.2
Tuna	0.5	20	2.5
Rainbow trout	0.5	15	3.4
Pacific halibut	0.4	17	2.3
Atlantic cod	0.3	43	0.7
Alaska King crab	0.3	38	0.8
Dungeness crab	0.3	30	1.0
Shrimp	0.3	27	1.1
Catfish	0.3	7	4.3
Haddock	0.2	29	0.7
Scallops	0.2	25	0.8
Northern lobster	0.2	22	0.9
Flounder	0.2	20	1.0
Red snapper	0.2	17	1.2
Sole	0.1	8	1.2

An iron deficiency is easy to fix since, once you're over 50, you only need about 8 milligrams (mg) a day. Fish, meat, and poultry supply loads of iron for busy lifestyles. Serve fish with a side of beans to up your iron. The iron in animal foods helps your body absorb the iron from plant foods like legumes.

Be tough with B6. This nutrient knows how to work. It has a hand in building red blood cells, proteins, and even brain chemicals. It regulates your blood sugar and fortifies your immune system. In short, vitamin B6 helps you stay hardy. Lucky for you, it's plentiful in protein-rich foods like fish. That makes it easy to get your quota of 1.5 mg a day for women over 50, and 1.7 mg for men over 50. Three ounces of fresh yellowfin tuna gives you about half this recommended amount. On your off-fish days, be sure to include a variety of B6-rich foods like bananas, prunes, potatoes, and spinach, or an occasional serving of lean meat such as turkey or chicken breast.

Bet on B12. Now that you're supplying your body with all those important omega-3 fatty acids, you need vitamin B12 to put them to good use. This member of the B family also works closely with its cousin, folate, to make red blood cells. What's more, it protects your nerves and is a vital part of many natural body chemicals.

If you're over 50, your B12 bill totals 2.4 micrograms every day. That may not sound like much, but your body has a harder time absorbing it from food as you age. As a result, B12 deficiencies are common among older adults. That's why experts recommend you pay close attention to meeting your needs for this nutrient. Animal foods, particularly fish, shellfish, and red meat are bursting with it. Clams, crab, salmon, sardines, trout, and tuna, in particular, are top-shelf sources. Fortified cereals add their own share to the mix.

Fish is also a storehouse of protein; key trace minerals, including selenium, copper, fluoride, and iodine; and major minerals like calcium, potassium, phosphorus, and magnesium. The list goes on, but you get the point. Let fish grace your plate two or more times a week for all these protective benefits.

Dangerous fish: how to stay off the hook

If fish is so good for you, why don't more people eat it? Maybe because they're worried about pollutants. When you serve up fish, you also risk eating the toxins — like mercury, PCBs (polychlorinated biphenyls), and dioxin — they've absorbed from polluted lakes, streams, and oceans. The older and larger the fish, the more pollutants it may contain. That's because big fish get bigger by eating other fish, which also contain toxins. For example, white, albacore tuna has about twice the mercury levels of light tuna, which comes from smaller fish.

Safe seafood shopping

Buy your seafood from a seller that works hard at food safety, and you'll help protect your family from the risk of food poisoning. Use these tips from the FDA to help you choose.

▶ Notice how the fish are displayed. They should be in a case or under protective cover — and should literally be "on ice." Their ice bedding should be thick and show no signs of melting. What's more, each fish should be displayed belly down so that the ice drains away from it.

▶ Check that employees are wearing clean clothing and a hair covering.

▶ Watch to see whether employees wear disposable gloves to handle the fish and whether they change gloves after handling raw seafood.

Don't let the fear of pollutants turn you into a landlubber. Most people don't eat enough fish to be in serious danger. The American Heart Association says the health benefits of eating fish twice a week far outweigh the risks for older men and postmenopausal women. According to the Food and Drug Administration, most people are safe eating up to 12 ounces a week of a variety of low-mercury fish such as fresh tuna, red snapper, orange roughy, marlin, and others.

Whether shopping for fish or eating out, take the following measures to limit your mercury and PCB exposure.

▶ Avoid tilefish, shark, swordfish, and king mackerel.

▶ Choose fish lower in mercury. These include salmon, herring, sardines, shad, trout, mackerel, and whitefish.

▶ When cooking farm-raised salmon, grill or broil it to let the juices drip out, cook the fish until the internal temperature reaches 175 degrees Fahrenheit, and remove the skin before eating.

If you're an avid angler, knowing where to reel them in can keep you safe. Find out which rivers and lakes are full of contaminants and which bodies of water are clean, then plan a toxin-free fishing trip. Check local advisories about the safety of fish caught in local lakes, rivers, and coastal waters. Otherwise, eat no more than 6 ounces of fish caught from local waters, and eat no other fish that week.

Get a hold of your state or local gaming officials for up-to-date warnings, or contact the Environmental Protection Agency for the latest pollution warnings:

U.S. Environmental Protection Agency
Fish and Wildlife Contamination Program
1200 Pennsylvania Ave., NW
Washington, DC 20460
www.epa.gov/ost/fish

Incredible vitamin cuts complications

It plays an important role in preserving vision, fighting infections and bacteria, maintaining your skin, and healthy bone growth. Plus, it fights heart disease, cancer, memory loss, arthritis, respiratory distress syndrome, liver disease, Parkinson's, and complications of diabetes. Must be a multi-vitamin, right? No — just one super vitamin called C.

Are you getting 100 percent of the C you need each day? Japanese researchers found people with diabetes have lower levels of vitamin C in their immune cells than healthy people, and that diabetics with complications had even less C than those without.

That's a real problem if you have diabetes. Your cells produce renegade molecules known as free radicals as a natural part of normal body processes. Typically, you get enough vitamin C and other antioxidants from food to neutralize free radicals and keep them in check. But experts suspect this antioxidant defense mechanism stops working in people with diabetes, allowing free radicals to get out of hand. These rogue molecules damage cells and systems over time, leading to some of the serious vascular complications, like heart disease, that often develop.

You can fight back by eating more brussels sprouts and other high-C foods. As an antioxidant, this vitamin helps protect you from the serious side effects of diabetes, such as blindness, amputation, heart disease, stroke, nerve damage, and kidney disease. The boatload of vitamin C in delicious foods like sweet red peppers, strawberries, and broccoli can also help control your blood sugar level and improve insulin sensitivity. Citrus fruits, another prime C source, have an added benefit because the acid in those fruits slows down digestion and helps stabilize blood sugar. And that's not all. Here's what else C can do for you.

Protects your heart. Vitamin C may lower your blood pressure, improve blood flow, and shrink your risk of stroke. Because it's an antioxidant, it may fight cholesterol by preventing the low-density

59

lipoprotein (LDL or "bad") cholesterol from becoming oxidized and, consequently, more dangerous to your artery walls. Have a glassful of orange juice with your meals and start fighting heart-damaging free radicals.

Boosts immunity. You may never get cancer or have a heart attack, but you will catch a cold. Meet your needs for C, however, and your cold won't stick around long. This vitamin spurs your body's immune system into action so you can fight off germs. Although experts say vitamin C doesn't reduce the number of colds

10 super sources of 'C'	
Wondering where to find the most vitamin C? Look no further than these 10 foods.	
Sweet red pepper	226 milligrams (mg)
Papaya	188 mg
Broccoli, 1 cup cooked	101 mg
Strawberries, 1 cup	98 mg
Brussels sprouts, 1 cup cooked	97 mg
Green pepper	96 mg
Cranberry juice cocktail	90 mg
Orange juice, 1 cup chilled	82 mg
Kiwi fruit	71 mg
Orange	70 mg

you get, it does cut down on how long and how seriously you're sick. It can also cut your risk of developing pneumonia up to 80 percent. Just getting 200 mg of vitamin C each day, elderly pneumonia or chronic bronchitis patients had fewer symptoms and recovered more easily. That's less than two glasses of orange juice a day.

Crushes cancer risk. Cancer may be called "the Big C," but that title rightfully belongs to vitamin C, which looms large in the battle against the disease. This antioxidant vitamin mainly shields you from free radicals that can cause cancer. Studies indicate vitamin C may protect you from stomach, throat, lung, bladder, and pancreas cancers. Some C-rich foods like oranges also provide fiber, folate, flavonoids, and the carotenoid beta-cryptoxanthin – all dedicated cancer enemies.

Benefits bones and joints. Your body needs vitamin C to build collagen – a fiber that holds bones, teeth, and cartilage together. Experts say the vitamin C in those juicy treats seems to slow the damage of OA. It might even repair damaged cartilage. Vitamin C also helps keep the calcium in your skeleton from being reabsorbed into your blood. For a one-two knockout punch against osteoporosis, buy orange juice with calcium added.

Mends your memory. According to scientists at the USDA-ARS Human Nutrition Research Center on Aging, your brain needs antioxidants to keep sharp. Otherwise, its cells wear down after years of free radical bombardment. Your memory becomes a little fuzzier, just like the picture in an old television. The USDA experts believe antioxidants like vitamins C and E can fix free radical damage done in the past as well as prevent damage in the future.

Sprinkle on this spice to slash blood sugar

How would you like to control your blood sugar and cholesterol with a spice that's probably in your pantry right now? Cinnamon can help regulate your blood sugar, cut triglycerides, and lower total cholesterol, according to some studies. Plus, it relieves indigestion and fights food poisoning.

Historians will tell you that in the ancient world, people were dying for cinnamon – literally. Considered more precious than gold, Egyptians used it to preserve bodies after death. Cinnamon comes from a bushy evergreen tree whose inner bark is dried and used as a spice. This fragrant spice, wildly popular for its ability to perk up a pie, has a new role.

▶ It turns out cinnamon's active ingredient, a polyphenol compound called methylhydroxy chalcone polymer (MHCP), mimics the action of insulin in your body and helps control blood sugar levels.

▶ Many people with diabetes have higher blood levels of fats called triglycerides and LDL or "bad" cholesterol. Insulin partly controls these as well as your blood sugar, and studies showed cinnamon helped lower unhealthy levels of fat and cholesterol.

Safe, quick defrost secrets

To cut your risk of food poisoning, thaw chicken in the refrigerator, in cold water, or in the microwave. You can thaw a 4-pound chicken in the refrigerator in about 24 hours, but thawing cut-up parts only takes 3 to 9 hours.

Thawing in cold water is even quicker. Place the chicken in its original wrap – or a water-tight plastic bag – in cold water. Change water often. Thawing the whole chicken takes about 2 hours. For speedy thawing of raw or cooked chicken use the microwave. Thawing time will vary.

▶ People with diabetes also have a high amount of free radicals circulating in their bodies. Lab experiments showed cinnamon was effective in neutralizing these damaging molecules.

▶ Cinnamon can kill *E. coli*, a dangerous bacterium that can cause severe diarrhea and flu-like symptoms. *E. coli* likes to hide in partially cooked meats and unpasteurized foods, like fresh apple cider. When scientists added cinnamon to apple juice infected with a large amount of *E. coli*, the cinnamon destroyed more than 99 percent of the bacteria after three days at room temperature.

▶ For hundreds of years, the ancient Greeks and Romans used cinnamon for better digestion. Although scientists can't tell you how it works, it may have to do with the way cinnamon heats up your stomach. Whatever the reason, adding cinnamon to your meal could help relieve your discomfort if you have trouble with frequent indigestion.

The strongest evidence of its anti-diabetes effects comes from a recent Pakistani study of 30 men and 30 women with diabetes. People in the study took 1 gram, 3 grams, or 6 grams of cinnamon, in the form of cinnamon capsules, each day for 40 days. Other study participants took equivalent amounts of placebo. People taking cinnamon, regardless of the dose, saw several significant improvements. Their fasting blood sugar dropped 18 to 29 percent, while their total cholesterol levels fell 12 to 26 percent. Bad LDL cholesterol decreased by 7 to 27 percent, and triglyceride levels plummeted by 23 to 30 percent.

The positive effects of cinnamon linger. Even 20 days after stopping cinnamon treatment, people often maintained lower blood sugar, cholesterol, and triglyceride levels. You don't need mass quantities of cinnamon to reap its benefits either. Just 1 gram, or about one-half teaspoon, each day will do the trick. In fact, even smaller amounts probably help.

It's easy to add cinnamon to your diet. Sprinkle some on your oatmeal, cereal, toast, yogurt, apples, and other fruit. You can even use it to spice up your meats and vegetables, such as cooked carrots, winter squash, or sweet potatoes. Swizzle cinnamon sticks in your hot cider, coffee drinks, and juices to add a healthy benefit to your beverages.

Unlike prescription drugs, cinnamon doesn't seem to have side-effects. However, don't eat cinnamon oil. It can be toxic even in small amounts. And don't fill up on cinnamon buns, pies, and other high-calorie, fatty sweets made with the spice. Just make this delicious spice part of a healthy diet.

Hearty breakfast beats disease

Mom was right – breakfast is the most important meal of your day. That's because what you eat for breakfast may determine your future health. Start your mornings off right to avoid life-threatening illness.

Want to stay off prescriptions? Eat more whole-grain cereal to reduce heart disease, blood sugar, and weight. Having a bowl of cereal for breakfast seems to both lower blood cholesterol and cut down the amount of fat and cholesterol you eat throughout the day. Whole-grain cereals, in particular, slash LDL and total cholesterol and boost insulin control – benefits that refined grains don't boast.

Processing, or refining, makes the carbohydrates in grain easier to digest, so their sugar enters your bloodstream in a burst. This causes post-meal spikes in your blood sugar and insulin that, over time, can lead to type 2 diabetes. Fiber-filled foods like whole grains help prevent diabetes because they slow down the process of converting carbohydrates into glucose. Also, if you eat a high-fiber carbohydrate, your body will respond with less insulin than it would if you eat a low-fiber food.

Don't buy into fake brown breads

Never eat bread? That's just baloney. It's all in the type of bread you eat. But don't be fooled by misleading "whole wheat" labels. Brown bread can be just as unhealthy as white bread. To tell the good from bad, just check the label. "Wheat flour," "enriched flour," "7-grain bread," and "degerminated corn meal" sound fancy, but they aren't whole grains. Instead, look for foods with these whole grains first in their ingredient list: whole oats, whole wheat, whole rye, whole grain corn, oatmeal, brown rice, cracked wheat or bulgur, pearl barley, or graham flour.

And don't fall for extras. While it might be nice to have calcium or protein added to the bread, the most important ingredient in your bread is whole grain.

Whole grains digest slowly, and research shows their insoluble fiber improves your insulin sensitivity and may help stave off diabetes. Eating just three servings of whole grains a day can trim your type 2 risk 20 to 30 percent. It also slashes your risk of metabolic syndrome, a group of health problems that increase your risk of diabetes, heart attack, and stroke.

Cereals are especially good at warding off diabetes. Women in one study who ate more than 7.5 grams of cereal fiber per day were 36 percent less likely to develop diabetes than women who ate less than half that amount. And 7.5 grams is not a lot of fiber. A 1-ounce serving of bran flakes for breakfast will supply you with more than 8 grams of cereal fiber. In fact, you can actually eat a little more of a cereal that's high in fiber without harming your total carbohydrate count.

For the most nutritious cereal, choose one made from the whole grain that contains at least 5 grams of fiber per serving. Keep these hints in mind to get the most fiber-filled bang from every bowl you eat.

▸ The name on the front of the cereal box may be misleading, so you'll need to read more to find out what's really inside. The nutrition information on the side panel will tell you that Kellogg's Complete Wheat Bran, for example, has only 4 grams of insoluble fiber per serving. Post's 100% Bran contains about 7 grams. Yet, you'll find a whopping 12 grams in a similar-sized serving of Fiber One from General Mills.

▸ The more sugar in a cereal, the less room for fiber. Check the labels even on cereals designed to attract grown-ups – like multi-grain Smart Start and Sunrise, made from organic grains. Ounce for ounce, these contain more sugar than Frosted Mini-Wheats.

▸ Don't assume all varieties of one brand are the same. A serving of regular Cheerios contains 3 grams of fiber and 1 gram of sugar. But you'll get only 1 gram of fiber and 13 grams – that's over three teaspoons – of sugar in the same amount of Apple Cinnamon Cheerios.

▸ Pass on cereals that don't list fiber content, like Cocoa Puffs. They don't contain any fiber, and by law, the manufacturer doesn't have to list it. You may see the words "Not a significant source of dietary fiber" in smaller print.

▸ Read the labels to see what other nutrients are offered, but don't give up fiber for extra vitamins and minerals. Make the most of the nutrients your cereal does offer by drinking all the milk you pour over your cereal. Some cereals have vitamins and minerals sprayed on the outside. Don't leave them dissolved in the milk at the bottom of your bowl.

Battle high blood sugar with blueberries

Every now and then, a great food comes along that not only tastes good but is good for you, too. Blueberries are sweet, juicy, cute, delicious, and packed with all sorts of amazing health benefits – like vitamin C, fiber, calcium, and iron. Sprinkling a handful of blueberries on your morning cereal could help lower your blood sugar and sharpen your memory.

They've long been a favorite folk remedy for high blood sugar, but scientists only recently found their own proof. Blueberries lowered blood sugar levels about 26 percent in animal studies in Italy. Plus, they can help keep your mind sharp and even reverse some of the effects of aging. Exciting new studies at Tufts University in Boston suggest blueberry extract may improve memory, coordination, and speed tests.

You can probably thank their truckloads of antioxidants, and you can't do better than a serving of blueberries for antioxidant protection. Even in healthy people, molecules called free radicals are created in your body whenever cells turn oxygen into energy. And these molecules are out to destroy healthy cells. Given enough time and opportunity, free radicals cause all kinds of sickness – even heart disease and cancer. Luckily, nature provides a delicious antidote in blueberries.

Each little fruit contains the pigment anthocyanin, which gives the berry its blue color. But anthocyanin is also a potent antioxidant that hunts down and destroys free radicals. In fact, scientists at the USDA-ARS Human Nutrition Research Center on Aging discovered blueberries are so full of goodness that a half-cup serving has the same amount of antioxidants as five servings of peas, carrots, apples, squash, or broccoli.

You'll find members of the blueberry family throughout Europe and Asia, including England where they grow a distant cousin called bilberries. More than 40 varieties are native to North America. Grab

---

Savvy ways to save money

To save money when shopping for groceries, remember the word HALT — hungry, angry, lonely, and tired. Don't shop when you are feeling any of these. You'll make wiser choices when your appetite has been satisfied, you feel rested, and all is well in your world. Otherwise, you are likely to buy more of those "comfort foods" you think will make you feel better.

Shop alone whenever possible. With other family members along you are likely to make more impulse purchases. Take their preferences into consideration when making your list — not in the grocery aisle.

---

a handful of fresh or frozen blueberries for a tasty breakfast topping, energy-boosting smoothie, or sweet, simple snack.

A few cups a day keeps diabetes away

Over 200,000 people could avoid type 2 diabetes this year if they would just wake up and smell the coffee.

If your breakfast includes a steaming mug of java, you're well on your way to diabetes protection. This common eye-opener has opened the eyes of quite a few researchers with its uncommon powers.

Lower your risk. Long-term studies show that people who drink more than a few cups of coffee every day have a lower risk of developing type 2 diabetes. Research conducted in different countries yielded similar results.

▶ In a recent Harvard study, women who drank four to six cups of coffee a day cut their risk by 30 percent. That means about 200,000 people – or one-third of the 600,000 new cases of diabetes the National Institute of Diabetes and Digestive and Kidney Diseases (NIDDK) says will be diagnosed this year – could prevent diabetes if they just knew about the protective benefits of coffee.

▶ Swedish women who drank five to six cups a day lowered their risk by more than 60 percent.

▶ People who drank a whopping 10 cups or more a day benefited the most in a Finnish study. Women reduced their risk by 80 percent, while men lowered their risk by more than 50 percent.

All of these studies relied on questionnaires from the participants, so a direct cause-and-effect link could not be established. But the evidence remains very strong.

Let the pros explain. Just as you might appreciate coffee for different reasons – the aroma, the taste, that jolt of caffeine – scientists have different theories about what makes coffee tick.

Some think caffeine may help your body control blood sugar over the long haul as your tolerance for it builds. But coffee's real hero might not be caffeine at all. That honor could belong to chlorogenic acid, which helps regulate blood sugar. Coffee's high levels of antioxidants, mostly in the form of chlorogenic acid, may also improve insulin sensitivity by protecting your cells from damage.

Other ingredients, including magnesium, potassium, and niacin, could also play key roles in staving off diabetes.

Get the full scoop. Because caffeine hampers your body's ability to control blood sugar in the short term, some researchers strongly advise people with diabetes to avoid it.

Researchers from Duke University measured the effects of caffeine on 14 coffee drinkers with type 2 diabetes. Caffeine didn't make much of an impact on an empty stomach. But when these people had caffeine with their meals, their glucose levels shot up 21 percent and their insulin levels skyrocketed 48 percent.

Because of these surprising results, the researchers recommend diabetics cut back on caffeine or even eliminate it from their diet entirely.

Keep in mind the study was very small and used caffeine pills rather than coffee. Even so, it's probably wise to drink coffee in moderation if you already suffer from this condition.

Pour carefully. Keep the following tips in mind before filling your mug.

▶ Consider decaffeinated coffee, which still has chlorogenic acids but very little of the caffeine of regular coffee. Go easy on the sugar, too.

▶ Stick with filtered coffee. Boiled coffee, the kind you get with a French press coffee maker, might not provide the same benefits.

▶ Use common sense. Don't go overboard and substitute mass quantities of coffee for a healthy diet, exercise, weight loss, and other proven strategies to prevent diabetes.

You can enjoy a cup of coffee just about anywhere − including your favorite bookstore. When buying coffee to brew at home, buy only enough for a week, and store it in a cool, dark place to keep it fresh.

Start your mornings off right − and take a few coffee breaks throughout the day − to avoid type 2 diabetes.

Satisfy your sweet tooth naturally

Sugar can give fresh fruits their sweet flavor or sodas their syrupy taste. The difference is in the company it keeps. When you eat fruit, milk, or even grains, you get a little natural sugar alongside a healthy dose of vitamins and minerals, water, and perhaps fiber.

Commercial sweets, on the other hand, contain concentrated amounts of refined or added sugar, and lots of energy, or calories, but very few nutrients. You'll get quick energy and little else.

Most of the refined sugar you eat probably comes from processed foods such as sodas, cakes, cookies, candies, fruit drinks, and dairy desserts like ice cream. Manufacturers add this extra sugar to tempt your taste buds. Added sugar is a major health concern. Eating too much of it tends to edge nutritious foods out of your diet and contribute to both weight gain and tooth decay. Plus, foods with added sugar are often also loaded with saturated fat and cholesterol, prime suspects in many illnesses.

Say hello to the sweet life

People with diabetes can't eat sweets, right? Wrong. Too often, having diabetes can make you feel sentenced to a lifetime of bland food. Not so, says the American Diabetes Association.

You do need to watch what you eat, but as long as you work them into your meal plan the way you would other carbohydrates, you can eat sweets in moderation and still keep your blood sugar in line. That's because the total amount of carbs in a meal has a bigger impact on your blood sugar than the type of carb.

Most people with diabetes can eat three to four servings of bread, potatoes, pasta, or other starchy foods daily, in small portions. In fact, whole-grain starches boast lots of fiber, which keeps your digestive tract healthy. Desserts and sweets are OK, too, if you eat them in moderation, exercise regularly, and eat an overall healthy diet.

Unfortunately, most people get far more sugar than they need in a day, mostly from processed, prepackaged foods. Just 2 ounces of chocolate or a single 12-ounce cola may deliver more than 8 teaspoons of sugar, while half a cup of canned corn may pack another 3 teaspoons. Sweeteners like honey and molasses fare little better, providing almost no nutrients but plenty of calories. In fact, teaspoon for teaspoon, honey harbors more calories than white sugar. So what's a sweet tooth to do?

Eating a goody once in a while as a reward for hard work won't hurt most people. But indulging your sweet tooth too often can undo any fitness gains you make and send your sugar control into a nosedive, not to mention put on the pounds around your middle. Artificial sweeteners may offer one solution. Saccharin and aspartame, for instance, sweeten foods without adding extra calories. Unfortunately, some research links these sugar substitutes to headaches and migraines.

Crack the sugar code. Check ingredient labels for code words like corn sweetener, corn syrup, fruit juice concentrate, honey, syrup, invert sugar, malt syrup, molasses, table sugar, raw sugar, and brown sugar. Avoid foods that list a sugar among its first ingredients.

Heat it up for natural sweetness. Make low-sugar dishes and serve them warm. This makes many foods taste sweeter.

Add flavor, not sugar. Cook with sweet-tasting spices like allspice, cinnamon, nutmeg, or cloves.

Pick unprocessed products. Whole grains, fruits, and vegetables contain less added sugar than their processed, prepackaged counterparts. Many have a sweet taste anyway.

In fact, your best bet is to develop a taste for naturally sweet foods — whole grains and fruits like strawberries or blueberries — and eat them in place of snack foods high in added sugar. Try these tempting and nutritious treats.

▶ Make fruitsicles from puréed pineapple, mango, or other fresh fruits or juices. Pour into ice cube trays and freeze on wooden sticks.

▶ Slice a banana into thin, round pieces, then spread them flat on a cookie sheet. Cover and freeze for a frozen treat.

▶ Mix fresh or frozen fruit into a cup of low-fat yogurt, or add atop a whole-grain breakfast cereal.

▶ Quench your thirst with water rather than sugary sodas or fruit drinks. Add a dollop of unsweetened juice for flavor and a hint of sweetness.

Learn to spot hidden sugars

Want to avoid sugar? First, you'll have to find it, and that takes a little detective work. "Hidden" sugars can sabotage your healthy diet. Some foods, like fruits and milk, naturally contain sugar. Others, like sodas and ketchup, have sneaky sugar added during processing. Before you buy, check this list of foods that are surprising sugar sources.

▶ tomato paste

▶ popcorn, potato chips

▶ frozen waffles

▶ ready-to-eat pudding

▶ baked beans with franks

▶ nonfat yogurt

▶ unsweetened applesauce

▶ canned fruits like peaches, pears, pineapple, and cocktails packed in syrup

▶ fruit punch, cranberry juice cocktail, and other sweetened fruit juices

- frozen, sweetened strawberries, blueberries, and raspberries
- milk shakes
- condensed milk and evaporated milk
- frozen, sweetened juice concentrates

Names for sugar	What they mean
glucose (also dextrose), fructose (also levulose), galactose	types of monosaccharide sugars
lactose, maltose, and sucrose	types of disaccharide sugars
evaporated cane juice	a purified form of raw sugar
concentrated fruit juice sweetener	a syrup usually made from grapes and used to sweeten foods that claim to be "all fruit"
corn syrup and high-fructose corn syrup	concentrated sugars made from cornstarch
corn sweeteners	a mixture of corn syrup and sugar solutions made from corn
raw sugar	first crystals derived from processing, must be purified to be sold in U.S.
confectioner's sugar	99.9 percent pure powdered sucrose
brown sugar	white sugar with molasses added

You can spot the total amount of sugars – both added and natural – in any packaged food by reading the Nutrition Facts label. Manufacturers list the amount of sugar in their products below the total amount of carbohydrates.

Take your detective work a step further by reading the ingredient list. This list only includes sugars added during processing, and ingredients are listed in order of amount. For instance, foods that list a sugar as one of the first two or three ingredients contain lots of added sugar, so stay away from them. Don't be fooled by the fancy names, either. Sugar goes by many names, including those listed on the previous page.

The scoop on artificial sweeteners

Sugar free! No added sugar! Diabetic foods jump off grocery store shelves, making promises most of them can't keep. Anyone who has ever eaten a "sugar-free" snack and then watched their blood sugar skyrocket knows that navigating the maze of artificial sweeteners isn't easy.

Basically, sweeteners come in three types – regular, reduced-calorie, and low-calorie. Sugar, cane sugar, fructose, honey, brown sugar, molasses, and confectioner's sugar are regular-calorie sweeteners. Reduced- and low-calorie sweeteners are sugar substitutes or artificial sweeteners.

Reduced-calorie. Also known as sugar alcohols, this group includes all the "-ols" – mannitol, sorbitol, xylitol, lactitol, erythritol, and maltitol, as well as isomalt and hydrogenated starch hydrolysates. They often show up in "sugar free" or "no sugar added" foods like candy, gum, and desserts.

You may think that means they're "free" foods, but they're not. They still contain carbohydrates and calories – about half as much as regular sugar – so they still raise your blood sugar. Don't forget this important fact when snacking on foods made with reduced-calorie sweeteners. Otherwise, you'll be in for an unpleasant surprise.

When counting these carbs, the American Diabetes Association says to look at the Nutrition Facts panel on the food's label. Check the amount of carbohydrates from "sugar alcohols" and divide it by two. Subtract that from the total number of carbohydrates in the food, also under Nutrition Facts, to get the number of carbs you should count.

Low-calorie. Aspartame (NutraSweet, Equal), saccharin (Sweet'N Low, Sugar Twin), sucralose (Splenda), and acesulfame potassium (Sweet One, Swiss Sweet, Sunett), on the other hand, do count as "free." They boast no carbohydrates and no calories and won't raise your blood sugar, unlike reduced-calorie sweeteners.

Worries about the safety of aspartame and saccharin once dogged these sweeteners. But both the Food and Drug Administration and the ADA say years of extensive research proves they are safe to use in the small amounts you would add to foods and recipes. Aspartame, however, may cause headaches and even migraines in some people. If you're prone to headaches or suspect a link, try the side-effect-free, low-calorie sweetener sucralose (Splenda), instead. Also, people with the rare genetic disease PKU (phenylketonuria), which doctors screen for at birth, should limit their use of aspartame.

Fake sugar scoop

Be careful when trying reduced-calorie sweeteners. Your digestive system does not absorb them well, so they may cause diarrhea in some people.

Sweet substitutes take the guilt out of baking

Low-calorie sweeteners can let you bake your cake and eat it, too. But some sugar substitutes don't hold up to the heat of cooking and baking, and most can't be used as equal-measure replacements.

Sugar — whether it's brown sugar, white sugar, or raw sugar — does more for baked goods than simply make them taste sweet. It also makes foods moist, caramelizes and liquefies at high temperatures, and helps goodies last longer after baking. But you can probably reduce the amount of sugar in a recipe by about one-third without changing the taste and texture of your home-baked treats.

Some manufacturers of low-calorie sweeteners have developed recipes to help you use their products in cooking and baking. Check the box or company Web site. But if you want to try substituting low-calorie sweeteners in your own recipes, follow these guidelines for each type of sweetener.

Acesulfame potassium is a Sweet One. At 200 times the sweetness of sugar, this low-calorie option is a good choice for cooking or baking. It's best to use it along with granulated sugar. You can substitute six packets (1 gram each) for each quarter cup of sugar in the recipe.

Aspartame can't take the heat. This sweetener breaks down under high heat, so you can't use it for cookies or cakes. But you can try it in recipes that let you add sweetener after the cooking is done, like puddings or no-bake pies. Substitute six packets (1 gram each) for each quarter cup of sugar.

Saccharin bakes up nicely. You can cook with this low-calorie favorite, but its manufacturer suggests using it for no more than half the sugar in your recipes. Use six packets (1 gram each) for each quarter cup of sugar.

Sucralose makes an even trade. Granular sucralose is easy to use since you simply substitute it in equal measure — one cup for

Free recipes at your fingertips

Recipes, recipes, recipes! From sugarless apple pie to low-fat chicken soup, and even banana bread for diabetics. You can get them all for free by going on the Internet. Diabetes-friendly Web sites like these offer low-sugar versions of your favorite foods without charging you a dime.

▶ *www.diabetic-recipes.com*

▶ *vgs.diabetes.org/recipe/index.jsp*

▶ *diabetes.sd.gov/cookbook.htm*

▶ *allrecipes.com*

▶ *www.cooksrecipes.com/category/diabetic.html*

one cup — for sugar. Watch the clock when you're baking, however, since recipes made with sucralose tend to bake faster than with regular sugar.

Although you're saving carbs and calories when you substitute low-calorie sweeteners, don't forget you haven't replaced the fat in recipes. Indulge yourself wisely.

Beans: a truly 'magical' food

Beans are high in fiber (both soluble and insoluble), low in fat, and rich in protein. Known as the 50¢ meal, beans are the least expensive and best source of fiber, which helps keep a lid on cholesterol and blood sugar. They're also called the "poor man's meat" because they're a cheap way to get protein. These plate staples belong to the legume family, plants whose seeds develop in pods. Peas, lentils, peanuts, and soybeans do, too.

Most legumes are packed with vitamins and minerals, one of which could prevent diabetic neuropathy. Marked by tingling, burning, and numb hands and feet, it's a common problem for people with diabetes. But research suggests inositol, a powerful form of B vitamin found in legumes, can help prevent this painful condition.

Chronically high blood sugar damages your nerves over time, especially the protective outer "skin" called the myelin sheath that surrounds each nerve cell. As this protective sheath breaks down, so do the structures inside your nerves. Nerve signals may start going haywire, with some slowing down and others getting blocked. Experts think a shortage of myo-inositol, a form of this B vitamin, is one culprit behind diabetic neuropathy. In rats, a deficiency of myo-inositol leads to nerve damage similar to what people with diabetes experience. Feeding rats more of this B vitamin, however, seems to prevent this nerve damage and help nerve cells repair themselves.

Beans have a lot more to offer, though. If you're looking for a tasty way to get more zinc, try a little black bean soup. For extra iron, a small serving of navy beans will do the trick. Lima beans are particularly rich in potassium, while black-eyed peas are your best bet for magnesium. Whether you buy them dry or fresh, legumes could very well be your diet's best friend.

Switch them with meat. By providing plenty of protein without artery-clogging cholesterol and saturated fat, beans and other legumes make wonderful alternatives to meat. If you switch just half of your protein intake from meat to legume sources, you could lower your cholesterol by 10 percent or more.

Beans are also high in fiber, which can protect your heart and shrink your stroke risk, and have been shown to lower cholesterol. They may even help you lose weight without cutting calories. In fact, in one study, a group of healthy men didn't cut calories but

> **One serving of legumes means:**
>
> ▸ ½ cup tofu
>
> ▸ ½ cup beans
>
> ▸ 2 tablespoons peanut butter

added about two and a half cups of beans to their usual daily menu. They still lost weight. Substitute a cup of cooked legumes in place of meat twice a week.

Eat 'em whole. Building more beans, peas, lentils, and other legumes into your diet can help lower blood sugar as well as improve insulin sensitivity and glycemic control. But how you cook those legumes may be just as important as how many servings you eat.

Processing and milling legumes and grains breaks down the walls between individual plant cells, making it easier for your body to digest and absorb the starch in those cells. That puts sugar in your blood stream faster, leading to blood sugar spikes after meals.

Eating whole beans and grains may prevent that spike, because they break down more slowly. In fact, your body may not digest these unprocessed foods completely, so some of the sugar may never make it into your system. Plus, unrefined legumes make you feel full longer than their processed counterparts, so eating the whole beans could help you lose weight.

Be creative. You can eat legumes raw or cooked in any number of dishes. Cannellini beans, pea pods, and cooked fava beans are delicious when tossed into salads, while lentils and kidney beans are great for adding flavor and thickness to soups, stews, and chilies.

Knock the "wind" out of them. Despite their star quality, many people shun beans. Between their image as a food for poor people, and their ability to cause gas, beans have a serious public relations problem. However, you can eat beans and have friends, too. You can easily reduce the amount of gas legumes produce by changing the water a few times while you're boiling them. Another alternative is to add a product called Beano to legumes after cooking. A few drops is all it takes to make them "wind free."

Green tea: brew up powerful protection

Wouldn't it be nice if you could fight cancer, heart disease, type 2 diabetes, flu, even bad breath – just by sipping a steaming cup of tea? You can, if you make it green tea.

It is possible that green tea can rev up your metabolism, improve insulin sensitivity, regulate blood sugar and cholesterol levels, and decrease heart disease risk.

Excess glucose in your blood reacts with oxygen to produce free radicals, unstable molecules that wreak havoc, particularly on your blood vessels. If you have diabetes, you have more free radicals floating around than other people, more than your body can get rid of on its own. These extra free radicals are the main culprits behind the serious complications faced by people with diabetes, such as heart disease, kidney damage, nerve damage, and diabetic cataracts and vision loss.

That's where antioxidant-rich green tea comes in. It gives your body extra ammunition to disarm free radicals and, in the process, might protect you from developing diabetes complications. In a Japanese study, men and women who drank six or more cups of green tea a day were 33 percent less likely to get type 2 diabetes. Other teas, including black tea and Chinese oolong tea, didn't offer that protection.

Pour the perfect cup

You can find green tea in a variety of places, from specialty shops to your local supermarket. Although green tea bags are widely available, you might want to buy your tea fresh. Look for leaves that have an even color and a delicate, not strong aroma. Since top grades of tea are handpicked, you should see fewer stems in more expensive varieties.

Tea leaves of top-grade teas are also more tightly rolled than lower grade teas. This gives the tea a more consistent flavor. It also means a pound of high-quality tea will look smaller than a pound of lower-quality tea.

Steep green tea for 3 minutes in hot, but not boiling, water. Drink it before it cools and turns brown — a sign the antioxidants have stopped working.

The researchers think the caffeine in green tea may be partly responsible, but likely so are its rich stores of antioxidants known as catechins.

▶ In lab studies, green tea catechins protected diabetic red blood cells from oxidative damage. That's why experts think eating catechin-rich foods could help people with type 2 diabetes ward off long-term complications.

▶ Other research shows green tea improves how your body uses and stores glucose. These findings suggest it could prevent type 2 diabetes or lower your risk by controlling after-meal blood sugar spikes.

▶ For the same reason, green tea might also help treat high blood sugar in people with existing diabetes.

Experts say the Japanese custom of drinking green tea in small amounts throughout the day might be the secret to keeping antioxidants circulating in your body. So keep filling up that cup while you take a look at what else this potent brew can do.

Boosts your metabolism. It was almost as if they'd discovered how to rejuvenate their metabolism. A group of middle-age, obese women lost twice as much weight as others on the same diet after only two weeks. Their secret? They took green tea extract with meals, which totaled 1,800 calories a day. Scientists suggest antioxidants in green tea, called catechin polyphenols, could help burn more calories. Try the natural tea instead of the extract until more research tests the supplement's safety and effectiveness.

Crushes cancers. If cancer is a frequent visitor to your family tree, green tea might be your new best friend. Drinking five or more cups a day could give women a better chance of surviving breast cancer and make early-stage tumors less likely to spread to lymph nodes. More than eight cups a day, for postmenopausal women, might mean even extra protection. Overall, green tea drinkers are more likely to have types of cancer that respond to medical treatment, and are less likely to get cancer again than other women.

Other studies show this remarkable drink fights cancers of the stomach, colon, prostate, and skin. Savor the protection. Slowly drinking and holding green tea in your mouth for a few seconds at a time keeps high levels of antioxidants in your mouth and throat. Scientists believe this could be why green tea drinkers get fewer oral and esophageal cancers than other people. What a great reason to relax over a cup.

Heads off heart problems. While you linger over another cup, green tea gets to work lowering your blood pressure and cholesterol. That means less risk of heart attack or stroke. Heavy coffee drinkers might want to skip a few cups of joe in favor of this wonder liquid. A Harvard Medical School study found that tea drinkers had a lower risk of heart attack than java lovers. Scientists believe an amino acid in green tea, called theanine, is responsible for keeping blood less sticky so it can move smoothly through your arteries. Preventing plaque build-up this way can reduce your risk of heart disease, stroke, and other health problems.

Fights the flu. Teas contain protein markers that resemble those of bad bacteria, parasites, and fungi. Scientists think drinking tea regularly may prime your immune system to recognize and fend off these dangerous foreign invaders, maybe making you more immune to certain illnesses.

Banishes bad breath. Green tea may also guard your mouth by curbing the growth of bacteria that cause cavities, plaque, and bad breath.

Discover the secret to a super-long life

People in Mediterranean countries like Greece live longer and suffer fewer diseases than anywhere else on earth. And even though their cholesterol may not be that much lower, fewer die from heart disease or suffer from other chronic illnesses.

Their long, healthy lives have made them famous and given doctors a reason to celebrate. Now you can, too. Experts have devised an amazing Mediterranean food pyramid based on the traditional eating habits of people in this part of the world. Studies show it seems to protect you from heart disease and certain kinds of cancer. It's also easy to follow. You don't have to make any drastic diet changes like cutting out all fat or carbohydrates. You can still eat pasta, cheese, even red meat. The key lies in moderation and in eating lots of whole, unprocessed foods.

The traditional Greek diet is full of fibrous fruits and vegetables, unrefined carbohydrates from whole grains and legumes, and heart-healthy monounsaturated fats from olive oil. At the same time, Greeks tend to get less saturated fat from animal foods. The result is an eating plan proven to lower LDL cholesterol and ward off heart disease.

Plants – not animal foods – make up the main part of Mediterranean meals. A plate heavy with fresh fruits, legumes, simple vegetables, and whole-grain pastas and breads sits in the middle of this healthy table. Some experts believe the nutrients in these whole plant foods – fiber, antioxidants, and unrefined carbohydrates – lend the Mediterranean diet its protective effects. Start eating like you're in the Mediterranean to protect yourself against diabetes, heart disease, and cancer.

Pick lots of produce. Put a variety of fruits and vegetables at the top of your grocery list, and eat between seven and 10 servings of them each day. Lay off the heavy cream and butter sauces. Opt instead for steaming or stir-frying vegetables in olive oil.

Go for the grains. Add whole-grain breads, cereals, and other unrefined grains like brown rice, couscous, bulgur, or polenta for a hefty dose of fiber. Avoid refined grains such as white bread, biscuits, and sweet, buttery baked goods.

Buy into beans. Make legumes and tree nuts a regular part of your day. Soybeans, peas, lentils, and other beans are top-notch legumes, while walnuts, almonds, and pecans are excellent nut choices. Just stay away from the salted and honey-roasted varieties.

Eat, drink, and be merry

According to the Journal of the American Medical Association, a combination of the Mediterranean diet, moderate exercise and drinking, and no smoking can lower mortality rates by 65 percent.

Land more fish and chicken. Fish are particularly kind to your heart and may account for the unusually good health people on the Mediterranean diet enjoy. Fatty fish like salmon, trout, and herring supply you with much-needed omega-3 fatty acids, a type of polyunsaturated fat. In addition, work in an occasional serving of skinless, low-fat poultry during the week.

Reduce the red meat. Plan beef and other red meats as a treat a few times a month. Skip fatty or processed meats like sausage and bacon, and limit your eggs to just a few each week.

Decrease your dairy. If you lived in the Mediterranean region, you might not have access to cow's milk every day. Greeks tend to eat yogurt and cheese made from goat and sheep milk, which has a stronger flavor, so a little goes a long way. In fact, while Western diets emphasize dairy products for bone health, Greeks eat dairy more sparingly. This also cuts back on the saturated fat in their diet. You can keep your dairy by choosing low-fat versions such as skim milk and nonfat yogurt whenever possible. But learn to skip high-fat ice cream, cheese, and whole milk.

Load up on olive oil. To the Greeks, it's as good as gold. People from this part of the world often use it in place of other cooking oils, fats, butter, and dressings — and research suggests you should, too. Studies prove the monounsaturated fats in olive oil lower LDL and raise HDL cholesterol, clearing fat deposits out of your arteries and lowering your risk of heart attack. It's not enough, though, to simply add olive oil to your diet. You need to use it instead of harmful saturated and trans fats like butter, margarine, shortening, lard, and corn oil. Extra virgin olive oil is the best kind. Make the switch, and you could be singing a happy 100th birthday to yourself.

Watch out for other fats. Saturated and trans fats pose an alarming threat to your health. Luckily, they make up only a small amount of the energy, or calories, you eat each day on the Mediterranean diet. Cutting back on fatty meats; replacing butter and other fats with olive oil; and building meals out of whole, unprocessed plant foods goes a long way to putting a lid on saturated and trans fats in your diet.

Snack on fewer sweets. Sweet snacks and sugary or fattening desserts are the exception, not the rule, in a Mediterranean meal. You can enjoy them a few times a week as special treats, but try making fresh fruit your regular dessert.

Magnesium: a 'magical' mineral for diabetes

Generations of philosophers have been stumped by one simple question: Which came first, the chicken or the egg?

Scientists studying type 2 diabetes and magnesium deficiency face a similar riddle. Does diabetes cause magnesium deficiency or does magnesium deficiency help cause diabetes? Whatever the answer, scientists agree on one thing — it's important to get enough of this "magical" mineral, since it seems to help prevent diabetic complications such as heart disease, eye disease, kidney disease, and high blood pressure.

Evidence shows that people with diabetes are more likely to be lacking in magnesium. This could be due to increased urination because of abnormal blood sugar levels and the effect of insulin on

Fresh is best

Your best bets for more magnesium — shop for fresh and organically grown foods. Processing removes this precious mineral, and experts say organic produce contains much more magnesium than conventionally grown vegetables.

the body. Diabetes-related kidney disease also may worsen magnesium problems.

If you are low in magnesium, you will have a harder time processing carbohydrates, be more open to insulin resistance, and may suffer high blood pressure, irregular heartbeat and other heart problems, and possibly eye problems. Scientists think you could experience a vicious cycle where diabetes leads to magnesium deficiency, which in turn aggravates your diabetes.

But researchers also think magnesium deficiency may be an important factor in causing diabetes, not just something that affects the progress of the disease. So getting enough in your diet may help you avoid diabetes as well as keep you healthier if you get it.

Observational studies of magnesium intake and clinical trials of supplements show magnesium may help both prevent and treat diabetes.

▶ Harvard researchers tracked 85,060 women for 18 years and 42,872 men for 12 years. Those who got the most magnesium into their diets were one-third less likely to develop diabetes than those who got the least.

▶ A Simmons College study of 219 women without diabetes showed that women whose diets contained the most magnesium had lower fasting insulin levels than those whose diets had the least. Lower insulin levels mean greater insulin sensitivity, which can reduce the risk of diabetes.

▶ A Mexican study showed magnesium supplements help diabetes sufferers with low magnesium levels. After 16 weeks of taking 2.5 grams of magnesium chloride a day, people in the study boosted the concentration of magnesium in their blood and improved their insulin sensitivity.

In spite of these and other positive studies, it's too early to make a definitive call on magnesium. More clinical trials of magnesium-rich foods and supplements will help.

In the meantime, are you getting enough? Many people don't. Intake is especially low among black people. The Recommended Dietary Allowance (RDA) of magnesium for men 51 years and older is 420 milligrams (mg). For women the same age, the RDA is 320 mg. Foods should provide all the magnesium you need. Good sources of magnesium include avocados, nuts, legumes, whole grains, dark leafy greens, seafood, squash, baked potatoes with skin, broccoli, oatmeal, coffee, tea, and chocolate.

We may never unravel the chicken-or-egg riddle, but magnesium's role in diabetes treatment and prevention should someday become clearer. Until then, try adding more magnesium-rich foods to your diet.

"Silly" solution for high blood sugar

You've probably heard of using psyllium (pronounced "silly-um") to stay regular. But this soluble fiber found in Metamucil and other bulk laxatives also helps regulate your blood sugar and cholesterol levels. With that kind of one-two punch, psyllium can help knock out diabetes.

Slow and steady wins the race. That's the secret of psyllium's success. Technically an herb derived from the husk of psyllium seed, psyllium forms a gel that slows the digestion of food as it moves through your system. Because it takes longer to break down carbohydrates and absorb glucose into your bloodstream, insulin has more time to convert that glucose into energy. Psyllium likely lowers cholesterol by decreasing the absorption of fat and cholesterol, increasing bile acid, and inhibiting production of cholesterol by the liver.

Studies have yielded some pretty amazing results. Here are just a few examples.

▸ This one natural substance lowers LDL cholesterol as much as 13 percent and blood sugar levels by up to 20 percent.

These eye-popping numbers come from a study by the
Veterans Affairs Medical Center at the University of
Kentucky in which 34 diabetic men took 10.2 grams of psylli-
um a day for eight weeks.

▸ A Spanish study of 12 men and eight women with diabetes
reported encouraging results as well. After taking 14 grams of
psyllium a day for six weeks, they saw their glucose absorption
decrease by 12 percent. However, results varied greatly between
individuals. Their total cholesterol (7.7 percent) and LDL cholesterol (9.2 percent) also dropped significantly.

▸ Dozens of clinical trials have shown psyllium lowers total and
LDL cholesterol. In fact, the mountain of evidence convinced
the FDA to approve the following health claim: "Diets low in saturated fat and cholesterol that include soluble fiber from
psyllium seed husk may reduce the risk of heart disease."

▸ Not all studies are positive. Adding 1.7 grams of psyllium to a
serving of pasta did not have any effect on insulin or glucose in
an English study.

It's not hard to get psyllium into your diet. Besides Metamucil
and bulk laxatives, you can find it as a food additive in breakfast
cereals, such as Kellogg's Bran Buds. Or you can buy your own
psyllium at a whole foods store and sprinkle it on your morning
cereal. If you have diabetes, taking just one teaspoon, or about 5
grams, with water three times a day before meals can help reduce
blood cholesterol levels and control blood sugar levels.

Psyllium can interact with many medications, and some people
shouldn't take it at all. So talk to your doctor before supplementing
your diet with psyllium. If she gives you the green light, follow her
instructions very closely.

Also, be sure to monitor your blood sugar carefully while using
psyllium. Its ability to lower blood sugar means that it may push
blood sugar down too far in some people, especially when taken
with drugs that reduce blood sugar.

Psyllium has no other serious side effects. Just make sure to drink plenty of water. As with any fiber, don't add too much of it to your diet too quickly. Otherwise, you might experience bloating or diarrhea.

A-plus way to protect your eyes

Poor control of your blood sugar can damage the small blood vessels in your retina and lead to blurred vision and blindness. This complication of diabetes, called diabetic retinopathy, is the most common cause of blindness in adults, making people with diabetes 25 times more likely to become blind than other people.

Diabetes causes your eyes other problems, too, including a greater risk of certain types of cataracts. This clouding of the lens in your eye can leave you with cloudy or blurred vision, problems seeing halos or haze around lights, poor color perception, and sensitivity to light.

Luckily, there's hope, because when it comes to helping your vision, vitamin A gets an A-plus for protecting vision, especially for people with diabetes. It acts as an antioxidant, shielding your retina from free radical damage that can lead to macular degeneration,

Easy way to score an 'A'

Getting your daily vitamin A is simple. A single, medium-sized sweet potato gives you 1,096 micrograms (mcg) of vitamin A, more than the 900 mcg a day the government recommends for men over 50, or the 700 mcg suggested for older women. It has a moderate GI value and is heart-friendly, too, with no saturated fat or cholesterol, but lots of vitamin C.

cataracts, night blindness, and other vision problems. Even people with normal eyesight apparently benefit from getting more vitamin A in their diets, with considerably improved night vision and after-glare vision.

That's not all vitamin A does. Its antioxidant powers make it a valuable weapon against cancer and heart disease. It helps control your insulin levels if you have diabetes, protects you from ulcers, guards your mental abilities, and boosts your immune system.

People with diabetes tend to become deficient in this eye-saving nutrient. And since vitamin A depends on fat for absorption, so can people on very-low-fat diets or who have any disorder that interferes with fat absorption (such as celiac sprue).

Don't go overboard, though. Too much A can be toxic. It's probably not a good idea to take supplements, especially when you can get plenty of it through your diet. Meats and dairy products are loaded with vitamin A, but your body can turn plant compounds called carotenoids — such as beta carotene, lutein, and zeaxanthin — into vitamin A as well. Choose bright yellow or orange fruits and vegetables like apricots, carrots, and sweet potatoes for beta carotene. Green, leafy vegetables like spinach and collard greens give you plenty of lutein and zeaxanthin.

Caught early, diabetic blindness is preventable. An eye doctor (ophthalmologist) can spot the beginnings of diabetic retinopathy and other vision problems. You can even get financial help. The Diabetes EyeCare Program offers free exams and one year of care for people with diabetes. You must be at least 65 years old and a U.S. citizen or legal resident. Also, you can't be receiving health care through an HMO or the Veterans Administration. For more information, call 800-272-EYES (3937).

Put the pep in your step with biotin

Do you feel tired and sluggish, even though you're not sick? Maybe you need more B vitamins. One in particular, biotin, helps your health in all kinds of ways – especially if you have diabetes. It helps digest fats and carbohydrates, which is important for people with diabetes. Plus, it plays an important role in energy metabolism, growth, and the production of fatty acids and digestive enzymes.

It may even reduce the amount of insulin your body needs. A biotin deficiency keeps your body from using glucose properly, and studies have shown type 2 diabetics tend to have lower biotin levels than non-diabetic people. Animal studies found upping biotin intake increased insulin secretion, which would help lower blood sugar levels.

Biotin belongs to a whole family of high-energy B vitamins. These nutrients don't actually supply energy directly to your body. Instead, they act as co-enzymes, helping unlock energy-producing fuel from the food you eat.

Active forms of the B vitamins thiamin, riboflavin, niacin, pantothenic acid, and biotin all help release energy from carbohydrates, fats, and protein. Vitamin B6 assists in converting amino acids into protein, and vitamin B12 and folate are important in building and repairing new cells, particularly red blood cells.

B vitamins might help you feel better and have more energy in a matter of weeks. You can bite into more biotin by eating peanut butter, cereals, legumes, and nuts. Foods that supply the other B's include meat, dairy products, whole grains, nuts, and leafy green vegetables. If you still think you aren't getting enough, ask your doctor if you should take a B-complex supplement.

B vitamins for breakfast				
Ready-to-eat cereal	**Amount per cup**			
	Thiamin	Folate	Vitamin B6	Vitamin B12
General Mills Whole Grain Total	2.8 mg	1076 mcg	3.8 mg	8.6 mcg
Kellogg's Special K	.5 mg	676 mcg	2 mg	6.1 mcg
Kellogg's Complete Wheat Bran Flakes	2.1 mg	909 mcg	2 mg	8 mcg
Kellogg's Product 19	1.5 mg	676 mcg	2 mg	6 mcg
General Mills Total Raisin Bran	1.5 mg	673 mcg	2 mg	6 mcg
RDA for men over age 50	*1.2 mg*	*400 mcg*	*1.7 mg*	*2.4 mcg*
RDA for women over age 50	*1.1 mg*	*400 mcg*	*1.5 mg*	*2.4 mcg*

Reap the benefits of chocolate

Lower high blood pressure and help control diabetes – with chocolate? That's right. You can soften up those hard arteries and improve your insulin sensitivity with this flavorful favorite. It's probably in your kitchen right now.

A steaming mug of hot cocoa or a luxurious dark chocolate bar may sound decadent, but these tempting treats just might help you fight diabetes and heart disease.

Chocolate is a plant food, made from the cocoa bean found in the fruit pod of the cacao tree. Dark chocolate gets its heart-healthy benefits mainly from antioxidant compounds called flavonoids, like catechin and epicatechin.

These heart-healthy compounds cause your blood vessels to release nitric oxide, a chemical that relaxes vessels and lowers the pressure inside them. That's great news for your heart, because it means lower blood pressure. And new research shows it's equally great news for insulin problems. Having more nitric oxide floating around your bloodstream seems to improve insulin sensitivity and decrease insulin resistance.

Studies suggest flavonoid-rich dark chocolate or cocoa powder may help:

▶ improve insulin sensitivity and lower insulin resistance.

▶ increase blood flow.

▶ lower blood pressure.

▶ thwart free radical damage to LDL cholesterol, which helps prevent clogged arteries.

▶ inhibit blood clots.

▶ squelch inflammation.

▶ make arteries more flexible and able to dilate, or widen.

Clinical studies also suggest that chocolate does not raise cho-lesterol. "The fat in chocolate (cocoa butter) contains approximately 35 percent oleic acid — the monounsaturated fat found in olive oil — and 60 percent saturated fat, which is 35 per-cent stearic acid and 25 percent palmitic acid," says Mary Engler, Ph.D., a School of Nursing professor and vascular physiologist at the University of California at San Francisco. Scientists think the cholesterol-raising effects of palmitic acid may be offset by stearic and oleic acid.

Dark chocolate even provides important nutrients such as magne-sium, copper, and potassium. Plus, it's rich in antioxidants. A review of the research on chocolate and cocoa verified that antioxi-dants in chocolate flavonoids might help prevent free radical damage. What's more, researchers comparing the antioxidant con-tent of cocoa, tea, and red wine were surprised to find that cocoa has the highest levels.

So far, most studies are too small or too brief to prove that choco-late works safely for everyone over the long-term. Scientists say this field of research is still young, and more work needs to be done. Take these tips into account to get the most health benefit from these delicious indulgences.

Eat the right kind. Milk chocolate has much fewer flavonoids than dark chocolate, and white chocolate has nearly none, so don't expect them to deliver the same benefits. Even dark chocolates are not all the same.

Cocoapro, the cocoa in Dove dark chocolate, is specially processed to retain more flavonoids. It may be the one brand of chocolate that's actually good for your heart. When buying chocolate, look for the Cocoapro logo. A new Cocoapro product, CocoVia, is available in the health food section of many grocery stores; by calling 866-262-6266; or by going online to *www.cocovia.com*. CocoVia snacks contain cholesterol-fighting phy-tosterols as well as 100 milligrams of healthy flavonoids.

Enjoy in moderation. According to one study, you need around 125 grams (g) — about 4.25 ounces — of flavonoid-rich chocolate daily to get heart-healthy antioxidant benefits. The insulin study saw results with just 100 g of dark chocolate, roughly 3.5 ounces. Don't eat more than one or two small bars a day. Chocolate has plenty of fat and calories — just 100 g packs more than 500 calories, depending on the brand. Gaining weight is bad for your heart and diabetic control.

Snack on other sources. To help keep your flavonoid levels from tapering off, try eating other foods rich in the same flavonoid as chocolate. Good choices include green and black tea, sweet cherries, apples, purple grapes, blackberries, red wine, and raspberries.

Super food for heart and eyes

People eat 900 times more broccoli today than they did 25 years ago. Perhaps it's because this "crown jewel of nutrition" is one of the healthiest foods you can buy. Ounce for ounce, broccoli has more than twice as much vitamin C as oranges. It's also a good source of four vitamins and minerals that can help diabetics avoid poor circulation, clogged arteries, and even cataracts — folate, vitamin A, potassium, and calcium. Plus, this member of the cabbage family packs several phytochemicals that help prevent disease.

Keeps vision keen. You want to keep the world around you sharp and clear for as long as possible. That's why you should start protecting yourself against cataracts and age-related macular degeneration right now. One way is to make sure broccoli is on your shopping list. This cruciferous vegetable is loaded with lutein and zeaxanthin, two carotenoids your body converts into vitamin A, which in turn may lower your risk of developing both these vision thieves. According to research, broccoli and spinach are the best foods for the job and the more you eat, the greater your protection.

Thrifty tips for buying broccoli

Use these tips to help you get the most value when you buy broccoli.

▶ When you buy expensive fresh vegetables, be sure you use every part you can. Broccoli stems can be peeled and cut into small strips, then cooked with the broccoli florets. Eat as is or purée in a blender to add to soup stock.

▶ If your recipe calls for just a few broccoli or cauliflower florets, buy them in the supermarket salad bar. You won't have left-over parts that might go to waste, and you'll save preparation time as well.

Bolsters heart health. Vegetables are good for your heart because they're low in fat and have no cholesterol. But broccoli, in particular, is one of the superstar heart protectors because of its well-rounded nutritional qualities. It's rich in folate, a B vitamin that fights the artery-damaging amino acid homocysteine, and it's jam-packed with natural chemicals called flavonoids. These protect your blood and arteries from clotting, oxidation, and inflammation.

A 10-year study of more than 34,000 post-menopausal women found those who ate foods high in flavonoids reduced their risk of fatal heart attack by one-third. You need to eat broccoli or other brightly colored vegetables several times a week to get this heart-saving benefit.

Balances out blood pressure. Think sodium and think high blood pressure. Think broccoli and think potassium, calcium, vitamin C, and magnesium, four of the "good guy" nutrients that help control blood pressure. The famous DASH diet, sponsored by the National Heart, Lung, and Blood Institute and the National Institutes of Health, is designed to bring blood pressure – and the risk of heart disease and stroke – down. To do that, it recommends eating whole foods chock-full of these good guys.

16 tips to trim your grocery bill

Cynthia Yates has a knack for saving. She has written four books on how to budget, including *1,001 Bright Ideas to Stretch Your Dollars,* and her latest, *Living Well on One Income*. In fact, her thrifty tips could trim your grocery bills by as much as $50 to $150 a month, without cutting back on food. Eat well and be well, with these grocery secrets that save you money every day.

▶ Learn prices so you know a good deal when it comes your way.

▶ Get to know your grocers. "Talk to produce managers, stocking clerks, butchers, and store managers," Yates says. Ask questions and you may find out about special deals.

▶ Check the shelf price tag. It usually lists the price per pound or ounce, which can help you compare the cost of similar products.

▶ Bend and squint to find the best deals. "The less expensive products," she says, "are usually on the lowest shelves."

▶ Buy items in bags rather than boxes if you have a choice. Bagged foods generally cost less.

▶ Consider going generic. "Generic or store brands are often just as good as the gourmet brands," Yates says. And they might be cheaper.

▶ Check the expiration date on dairy products and other perishable foods before you buy.

▶ Ask the store to break up bunches of produce so you can buy a smaller amount. There's no sense paying for more than you will eat.

▶ Weigh prepackaged foods like fruits, vegetables, and meat. They sometimes hold more than their label claims. Yates says, "You may find a 5-pound pack of spuds weighing in at 6 pounds."

▶ "Shop seasonally," she advises. "Prices drop when markets have an abundance of certain foods." Holidays and back-to-school seasons, for instance, have their effect — for better or worse — on store prices.

▶ Steer clear of the gourmet aisle and processed food. "You can rip your own lettuce, or cut your own cheese, or season your own drumstick," Yates says.

▶ Skip the junk food. "Back off on the stuff that isn't good for you in the first place," she advises. An occasional treat is OK, but too much can drain your budget and your health.

▶ Don't give in to impulse buys while shopping — or at least limit them to two or three items per trip.

▶ Avoid overbuying. "I believe everyone should have enough water and food stashed to get through a week or so, should an emergency come along," says Yates. But she discourages hoarding. One of her rules — buy only what you eat, and eat what you buy.

▶ Check the prices at checkout. "Mistakes happen," she warns. "Watch the register and check receipts." A checker may scan an item twice, or the sale price may not ring up.

▶ Don't live with inferior products. "Politely return," she says. "If you have purchased a product that has gone bad, or not held up within reason, take it back."

▶ Skip items on the end of the aisle. Setting items there makes you think they are a special deal. But they may not offer the best price. "Sometimes," Yates says, "a walk down the aisle will find something less expensive."

▶ Resist temptation. Grouping items together encourages you to buy more than one product — like putting salsa next to the chips, or caramel dipping sauce by the apples. Don't buy it unless you need it.

Dodge diabetes with vitamin D

Got milk? Then you might not get diabetes.

In a 10-year study of nearly 40,000 middle-aged and older women, frequently eating low-fat dairy foods reduced the risk of developing type 2 diabetes. Women who ate the most dairy were 21 percent less likely to get the disease than those who ate the least. Focusing on low-fat dairy products earned them even more protection – a 36-percent lower risk.

Men fared similarly well in a separate study. Out of more than 41,000 men studied for 12 years, men who got the most dairy every day were the least likely to develop type 2 diabetes, 23 percent less likely than men who got the least. What's more, for every extra daily dairy serving the men ate, their diabetes risk dropped another 9 percent. Once again, low-fat and skim milk granted the most protection.

Learn the why's. Experts suspect the calcium and magnesium in dairy foods might lower diabetes risk, while lactose and dairy protein could make people feel full longer, cutting back on the obesity that often leads to diabetes. You further slash your chances of becoming part of the diabetes epidemic just by increasing your intake of one important vitamin commonly found in dairy products.

Vitamin D-deficiency increases your risk for both type 1 and type 2 diabetes, as well as metabolic syndrome. Experts suspect low blood levels of this vitamin cause problems with the cells in your pancreas that make insulin, called beta cells. Studies show animals with too little vitamin D don't make enough insulin, and that people with D-deficiency or type 2 diabetes produce more insulin when they start getting more vitamin D. Too little D may also lead to glucose intolerance, which could harm both your insulin and beta cells.

Get protection. Upping your intake even a little could have a huge impact. Bumping up blood levels of vitamin D from 10 nanograms (ng) per milliliter (mL) to 30 ng per mL can make your cells a whopping 60 percent more sensitive to insulin. That makes vitamin D treatment more effective than metformin, one of the most common drugs for insulin resistance. What's more, 60 percent could be enough to reverse your glucose intolerance, say scientists. It also lightens the burden on your beta cells, which otherwise have to work overtime to make enough insulin to move glucose from your blood stream into your starving cells.

Aside from diabetes, this one powerhouse vitamin may protect against heart disease and rheumatoid arthritis and may help prevent at least 13 different types of cancer. But don't go diving into the ice cream yet. Studies say chowing down on high-fat dairy foods like sour cream, whole milk, cream cheese, and other cheeses won't drop your diabetes risk. Only low-fat dairy products – including skim and low-fat milk, yogurt, sherbet, cottage cheese, and ricotta cheese – seem to protect you.

Have your day in the sun. Can't stand the taste of milk? No problem. The best way to get more of this incredible nutrient may be strolling in the sun. Vitamin D is known as the "sunshine" vitamin because your body naturally makes it when ultraviolet B (UVB) rays from the sun strike your skin.

This helps explain why certain people are more prone to vitamin D-deficiencies. People in the Northeast don't get enough UVB rays from November through March to make vitamin D, for instance. Dark-skinned people have a harder time making this vitamin, because the skin pigment melanin acts like sunscreen, blocking UVB. And everyone absorbs less vitamin D with age.

In most parts of the United States, you'll get your daily vitamin D needs by strolling with the sun on your neck, shoulders, and back (without sunscreen) each day between 11 a.m. and 2 p.m. — 15 minutes a day in summer and 20 minutes a day in early fall and late spring. Dark-skinned people need twice as much sun. Other experts, including dermatologists, argue inexpensive vitamin D supplements are the safest way to boost blood levels. If you choose to play in the sun, follow these tips to get the "sunshine vitamin" safely.

▶ Avoid burning. The same UVB rays that make vitamin D also cause skin cancer. Limit your sun exposure to 20 minutes a day if you burn easily and tan poorly. More than that will not noticeably increase your D levels.

▶ Hold off showering, bathing, or swimming for an hour after being in the sun to give your body time to absorb the vitamin.

▶ Get your daily D from supplements if you have fair skin, are sensitive to sunlight, or take medications that cause light sensitivity.

▶ Shop for cereals, milk, butter, and margarine fortified with vitamin D.

▶ Angle to occasionally eat fatty, coldwater fish such as tuna, sardines, herring, and mackerel, all rich in this nutrient.

▶ Discuss vitamin D supplements with your doctor first if you take calcium-channel blockers or thiazide diuretics.

▶ Avoid getting more than 2,000 IU of vitamin D from food and supplements in a single day.

Tiny seeds fight disease

Discover the miracle healing seed that lowers blood pressure; reduces risk of stroke; and fights arthritis, heart disease, type 2 diabetes, stomach disorders, and even mental problems. Sound too good to be true? It's not.

Flaxseed does all of this and more. In fact, for more than 10,000 years, humans have used flax to improve their health and way of life. Flax is an herb high in the heart-healthy fat omega-3, which is unusual for a plant. Whether in the form of flaxseed oil, ground flaxseeds, or flax flour, this plant gives you a good amount of alpha-linolenic acid, a type of omega-3 fatty acid that lowers blood pressure and your risk for stroke. It's also rich in fiber, which helps improve your cholesterol levels.

People used to eat foods with about a 50/50 balance of both fatty acids your body needs – omega-3 and omega-6. But that was before food became mass-produced. Since omega-3 fats go bad quickly, food manufacturers replaced them with longer-lasting omega-6 fats and hydrogenated oils – oils with hydrogen added to make them more stable. Now food companies don't have to worry about their products spoiling too soon. But you have to worry about not getting enough omega-3 and possibly getting too much omega-6.

Some doctors think the epidemic of heart disease, high blood pressure, inflammatory disorders, mental illnesses, and even cancer in modern societies can be traced back to imbalances in essential fatty acids. Artemis P. Simopoulos, M.D., has spent decades studying how nutrition affects health. In her book *The*

The facts about flaxseed

You can buy flaxseed in health food stores and some grocery stores. Grind the seeds with a coffee grinder and use them immediately. Flaxseed is an intense source of fiber. One tablespoon can contain up to 2.2 grams. To avoid gas and indigestion, start with small amounts and add it to your diet gradually.

Omega Diet, Simopoulos explains why you should add omega-3 fats back to your diet.

"One of the most important findings to come out of the research program," she says, "is that our bodies function most efficiently when we eat fats that contain a balanced ratio of the two families of essential fatty acids – omega-6 and omega-3 fatty acids. The ratio in the typical American diet has been estimated to be as high as 20 to 1."

You can fight back by limiting omega-6 fats and adding more omega-3s with flaxseed.

▶ Cut down on omega-6 fats by avoiding fried foods and foods made with corn, cottonseed, and tropical oils.

▶ Crush or grind flaxseed before eating it. Otherwise, your body won't absorb all the nutrients as the flax passes through your system.

▶ Try mixing flaxseed into applesauce, yogurt, or hot breakfast cereal for a fiber-filled treat.

▶ Buy flaxseed flour or grind up your own for baking breads, muffins, cakes, or even pancakes.

▶ Pour flaxseed oil on salads or vegetables in place of butter. Don't cook with flaxseed oil, though, because it breaks down in high heat and could be harmful.

▶ Store whole flaxseeds in a container in the refrigerator for up to one year. You can keep ground flaxseed in a container in the fridge, too, but it may not keep for longer than four months.

▶ Buy flaxseed oil in small amounts and store in the refrigerator. It goes rancid quickly.

Now that you know the secret to getting more flax in your diet, read on to learn more about the benefits.

Dethrones diabetes. If diabetes runs in your family, and you eat a typical modern-day diet, your chances of getting this blood sugar disorder are high. Who says you have to? Researchers are finding that diet is as closely linked to diabetes as family history. It seems the more omega-6 fats you eat, the more likely you are to be overweight. You're also more likely to become resistant to insulin – a double whammy that sets you up for diabetes.

Omega-3 fats don't treat you so cruelly. In fact, they help you. When laboratory animals were fed a high omega-6 diet, no one was surprised when they got fat. But animals fed the same amount and calories of omega-3 fats weighed an amazing 33 percent less. That's the difference between a 150- and 225-pound person. Maybe you don't need to eat all that tasteless low-fat food to stay slim. Maybe you're just eating the wrong kind of fat.

Besides keeping you thin, this friendly oil also helps your blood sugar. When a group of people with insulin resistance were switched to omega-3 fats instead of omega-6, they got better. They had lower blood pressure, lower blood sugar, and less harmful fat floating in their blood.

Guards your heart. Omega-3 fats contain alpha linolenic acid (ALA), an ingredient that should be near and dear to your heart. Eating ALA-rich foods like flax can make your blood less sticky, which keeps it from clotting too fast and causing a blockage. It also helps keep your blood pressure down and your heart beating regularly.

The people who live on the island of Kohama, Japan have the longest life expectancy in the world and the lowest rate of heart disease. They also have very high levels of ALA in their blood. Coincidence? Scientists think not. Experts suggest you eat about four fatty fish meals a week and use a vegetable oil high in ALA like canola or flaxseed oil.

Soothes stomach problems. As a rule, Eskimos don't get inflammatory bowel disease because of all the omega-3 they get from eating fish. Fish oil can help if you have trouble with an irritated bowel. But you might not like the fishy aftertaste, burping, and bad breath that come with it. In many studies, people who were given fish oil capsules stopped taking them because of these side effects.

But flaxseed oil, with its mild flavor, can give you the same benefits as fish oil. So if you can't bring yourself to eat one more serving of fish, why not add this oil to a salad of dark green, leafy vegetables? You'll boost your omega-3 intake and soothe your intestines at the same time.

Eases arthritis pain. If you were born in Japan, chances are you would never get arthritis. So what do they know that you don't? They get lots of the same substance that keeps Eskimos healthy – omega-3. Having the right balance of fatty acids in your body can protect your immune system from breaking down and causing diseases like arthritis.

Dr. Donald Rudin, a Harvard-trained physician and medical researcher, believes immune disorders can often be traced to out-of-balance omegas in your body. He explains the effect of fatty acids on the immune system in his book *Omega-3 Oils: A Practical Guide.*

"Normally, the immune system is kept under control by the body's essential fatty acid-based regulatory system," he says. "But dietary distortions, especially a shortage of the omega-3 fatty acids, are now known to contribute to – or even prompt – the breakdown of the immune system."

Rudin recommends one tablespoon of flaxseed oil per day for a 100-pound person who is deficient in omega-3. He also suggests you take a multivitamin. If you have food allergies, though, you should start with less oil and gradually add more. But don't overdo it. Taking more than six tablespoons daily might actually make your symptoms worse.

Calms a troubled mind. Until about 100 years ago, many poor people got a disease called pellagra, which is Italian for "rough skin."

Besides dry, rough skin, they had ringing in their ears, exhaustion, and mental problems. It took a long time for doctors to figure out that these people were missing a B vitamin in their diets. When the vitamin was finally added to staple foods like rice, the disease became history. Or did it?

Pellagra may have returned in − of all places − wealthy countries where people eat highly processed foods. Sure, there are plenty of B vitamins in foods now, but your body also needs a certain amount of omega-3 acids to use them. You could be well fed but still malnourished. Some doctors think the high rates of mental illness wherever you find a modern diet proves this connection. One expert has even claimed to have successfully treated mental illnesses such as manic depression, phobias, and schizophrenia with one to six tablespoons of flaxseed oil daily.

The hidden powers of spice

One of the most truly amazing developments of recent years is the discovery of powerful concentrations of natural healing agents − like natural blood sugar regulators and cancer-fighting antioxidants − in ordinary spices, including many that are probably in your kitchen right now. Scientists are currently studying these three spices for their power to battle diabetes.

Fenugreek. One of the oldest medicinal plants, fenugreek shows promise in lowering blood sugar levels for people with type 1 or type 2 diabetes. The seeds are rich in a soluble fiber that might help by interfering with the way your body absorbs sugar from food. And fenugreek is packed with an amino acid that stimulates your pancreas to release insulin.

This exotic seasoning is found in curry powder, or you can buy the seeds separately. Some experts suggest eating 5 grams, about 1 1/3 teaspoons, of whole seeds daily. Watch your blood sugar closely if you take insulin or other diabetic medications, as adding fenugreek

Treat curry with caution

Turmeric, the main ingredient in curry powder, can aggravate gallstones and blockages in the bile duct. Skip it if you have a history of gallbladder problems or if you take blood-thinning drugs, like warfarin (Coumadin), since it can boost their strength.

could cause hypoglycemia (low blood sugar). Of course, talk to your doctor first.

Chili pepper. Adding a dash of cayenne pepper livens up food while dampening after-meal insulin spikes. Australian researchers seasoned the food of 36 people, who were overweight, with cayenne chili pepper. After four weeks of eating the spicy food, their insulin and blood sugar levels were measured. Daily doses of this spice evened out insulin levels and lowered blood sugar spikes after eating. People in this study added 16.5 grams, a little more than three tablespoons, of a cayenne chili spice blend to their meals each day.

Turmeric. Years of poor blood sugar control can lead to cataracts. But turmeric, the yellow spice in curry powder, can put the brakes on cataract growth. This pungent spice seems to protect your eyes from damage caused by high blood sugar. Use it to liven up rice, beans, and sauces. For the most benefits, add a dash of black pepper to your dish and drink a cup of green tea with your meal. You'll absorb up to 20 times more curcumin, the active ingredient in turmeric.

Bite into better sugar control

Do you have type 2 diabetes? Make sure you eat plenty of apples, skin and all. They contain the work-horse nutrient chromium that shuttles excess sugar out of your bloodstream and into your cells.

A crucial mineral for people with diabetes, chromium helps your blood deliver and use insulin, guarding your body against insulin resistance and hypoglycemia. In test after test, scientists found that people who get more chromium have greater control over their blood sugar levels and are less likely to suffer from diabetes. These tempting fruits are also full of soluble fiber, which helps slow down the release of glucose into the bloodstream.

Try dipping apple slices in low-fat or all-natural peanut butter for a burst of the B vitamin biotin, too. You can get more chromium naturally from dairy products, fish and seafood, liver, mushrooms, whole-grain products, fresh fruits, nuts, unpeeled potatoes, and black pepper.

Beat snack attacks with these safe treats

If you have diabetes, you may feel like your snacking options are severely limited. But one new ingredient and an old kitchen stand-by are making it safe for you eat a treat without upsetting your blood sugar.

Daytime snacks. Certain starches, known as resistant starches (RS), resist digestion, meaning your body cannot break them down completely. RS occurs naturally in food, but manufacturers can also make it out of cornstarch and add it to food to create tasty snacks that don't cause high blood sugar (hyperglycemia). Because RS digests very slowly, the glucose in it enters your bloodstream gradually, keeping your blood sugar stable. In fact, since your body can't completely digest RS, some of the sugar never even reaches your bloodstream.

Diabetic snack bars such as Glucerna and Choice DM contain RS, making it easy for people with diabetes to enjoy a between-meals treat without sending their blood sugar through the roof. Experts say eating one with breakfast may also dampen morning blood sugar spikes. But RS may have bigger, long-term benefits for people with insulin resistance. Researchers tested the effects of 30 grams (g) of RS daily for four weeks in 10 healthy adults and found that RS supplements improved insulin sensitivity up to 33 percent in all 10 people. Look for maltodextrin – the code word for resistant starch – in the ingredients list on food labels.

Nighttime snacks. Sleep soundly all night with just a spoonful of cornstarch. Raw, or uncooked, cornstarch (UCS) makes a great bedtime snack. It's a complex carbohydrate your body digests and absorbs slowly, providing a steady source of glucose for up to seven hours. Research shows eating UCS as part of a bedtime snack may protect you from overnight and morning bouts of (hypoglycemia).

That was the case for kids with type 1 diabetes who ate a bedtime snack made with two teaspoons of raw cornstarch in one study. Out of 51 kids, only six who ate the cornstarch had low blood sugar at midnight, compared to 30 kids who ate a regular snack with the same amount of carbohydrates. By the next morning, only nine cornstarch kids were hypoglycemic, compared to 21 who ate the regular snack. You can try this yourself by dissolving two teaspoons of raw cornstarch in a non-sugary drink, like milk or sugar-free soda, before bedtime.

You don't have to mix your own cornstarch drink, of course. Food manufacturers have jumped on board with nighttime diabetic snack bars such as Nite Bite, Extend Bar, and Gluc-O-Bar made with UCS. Experts say eating them before bedtime, during long bouts between meals, after exercise, and after drinking alcohol may help prevent hypoglycemia.

Keep in mind that none of these snacks is meant to treat emergency hypoglycemia because they don't digest fast enough. For advice on treating emergency episodes, see *Quick way to raise low blood sugar* in the chapter *The Next Defense: When diet and exercise are not enough.*

Fresh fruits round out a healthy plate

Fruits have a big place in any meal plan, but if you're aiming to avoid or treat diabetes, then they are even more important. These three fruits, in particular, show promise for diabetes.

Pick cherries for prevention. Looking for a sweet way to beat diabetes? Start with cherries. In a new lab study, researchers at Michigan State University put some mice on a high-fat diet and others on a low-fat diet. The high-fat mice quickly gained weight, developed fatty livers, and became glucose intolerant. Researchers then began feeding them anthocyanins, compounds found in cherries, in addition to their fatty food.

After eight weeks, these obese, glucose-intolerant mice had lost weight, lowered their cholesterol, raised their insulin levels, were more glucose-sensitive, and once again had healthy livers. The researchers used Cornelian cherries but say the more popular tart cherries should work, too.

Go ga-ga for guava. The Chinese have used the guava fruit to treat diabetes for many years, and now experts know it may lower blood sugar. Research also shows guava helps lower blood pressure, reduce LDL cholesterol, raise "good" HDL cholesterol, and even protect against heart disease. Hard to believe one humble fruit can do all that. Plus, it's loaded with good-for-you nutrients, including beta carotene, lycopene, potassium, and soluble fiber – and it packs more than twice as much vitamin C as an orange. Grab a guava and get on the bandwagon. Try guava jelly on your toast instead of grape or apple jelly for an offbeat treat.

See a strawberry sunrise. The vitamin C, fiber, folate, and potassium in a handful of strawberries can provide powerful protection against multiple diabetes complications such as cataracts, slow-healing

The difference with dried

Dried fruits make great snacks, but they tend to have more sugar than their fresh counterparts. Take this into account when trying to get more fruit into your diet. Otherwise, dried and fresh fruits are nutritionally the same.

wounds, and high cholesterol. A good thing, since you are 60 percent more likely to develop cataracts if you have diabetes, and the cholesterol problems common with this condition raise your risk for heart attack and stroke. Bring home a carton of fresh, juicy strawberries, or grow your own. They're delicious in salads, smoothies, desserts, or just as a snack.

Discover fats that fight disease

It's spelled f-a-t, but to many people, "fat" is a four-letter word. Dieters and health-conscious eaters avoid it like the plague. That's because eating too much fat contributes to obesity, heart disease, high blood pressure, cancer, diabetes, and other diseases.

However, your body needs some fat to stay healthy. Fats provide the raw materials for making hormones and bile and carry the fat-soluble vitamins – A, D, E, and K – in your bloodstream throughout your body. Fats also add to the enjoyment of eating by making food tender, tasty, and pleasant-smelling.

Almost all foods contain at least traces of fat. Nutritionists refer to fat as an energy-dense food. That's because it packs 9 calories per gram, as opposed to 4 calories per gram for protein or carbohydrates. All fats are equal when it comes to calories, but there are big

Fats at a glance

Kind of fat	Sources	Effect on cholesterol levels	Action plan
Saturated (solid at room temperature)	Meat, butter, lard, whole milk, cheese, palm kernel oil, coconut oil, chocolate	Raises both LDL and HDL cholesterol	Limit to no more than 7 percent of calories daily. Eat lean cuts of meat and use low-fat dairy products.
Polyun-saturated (liquid at room temperature)	Vegetable oils like corn, safflower, sunflower, sesame, soybean, cottonseed	Reduces both HDL and LDL cholesterol. Too much may increase cancer risk.	Use oils and soft margarine in moderation, keeping total fat at or below 35 percent of calories per day.
Monounsatur-ated (liquid at room temperature)	Olive oil, peanut oil, canola oil, nuts, avocado	Lowers LDL. HDL stays the same or may be raised in some cases.	Use freely up to 35 percent of total calories per day.
Trans fatty acids (solid at room temperature)	Margarines, vegetable shortenings	Raises LDL, lowers HDL	Reduce or avoid commercially baked products (breads, cookies, cakes) and fried foods from fast-food restaurants. Seek recipes that offer other cooking options.

differences in how they affect your health. Believe it or not, some fats are actually good for you.

Make room for MUFAs. Monounsaturated fatty acids (MUFAs) are no slackers. They lower LDL cholesterol – the bad kind that clogs your arteries – and boost HDL cholesterol, the good kind that whisks cholesterol to your liver and out of your bloodstream. Plus, they help fend off diabetes, arthritis, high blood pressure, and some cancers. They can even boost your memory.

Experts from the American Diabetes Association (ADA) recently came up with a delicious eating plan that centers on MUFAs. "We found that a diet rich in monounsaturated fatty acids led to improvement in HDL (high-density lipoprotein) cholesterol, triglycerides and, most importantly, diabetes control," says Dr. Abhimanyu Garg, a member of the ADA's expert panel. That means MUFAs could help manage your insulin and blood sugar levels and fight diabetes-related heart disease.

Olive oil is bursting with MUFAs, as are canola oil, avocados, and peanuts. Use these to replace some of the unhealthy saturated fats in your diet. Slices of avocado are a good substitute for cheese on a veggie sandwich, for instance. And instead of cream cheese, spread a little natural peanut butter (made from 100-percent peanuts) on your bagel.

Pile on the PUFAs. Like monounsaturated fats, polyunsaturated fatty acids (PUFAs) lower LDL cholesterol. One PUFA in particular, known as omega-3, could give you an edge against diabetes. Experts say omega-3-rich foods like fish may cancel out some of the negative effects of being overweight. A diet rich in it seems to help cells release insulin and boost the action of insulin in your body.

Obesity is a major risk factor for type 2 diabetes, but in countries where fish is common, extra weight does not increase the risk of diabetes. In fact, these fat, fish-loving countries have about the same diabetes risk as people in "skinny" countries. One study found eating

6 ounces (about two servings) of fish each week protected seniors from developing glucose intolerance.

Omega-3s also clear clogged arteries, keep blood cells from sticking together, and ease high blood pressure. Plus PUFAs reduce your risk of heart attack and stroke as well as help with arthritis, Alzheimer's disease, cancer, and depression. For heart-healthy omega-3 PUFAs, eat two servings a week of salmon, halibut, herring, mackerel, or other fatty fish. Flaxseed, flaxseed oil, canola oil, and walnuts are also excellent sources.

Despite all the good it can do you, remember – fat is still fattening. Don't just add more fat to your existing diet. Make sure to cut calories somewhere else. A good strategy would be to trim saturated fats, like red meat, cheese, and butter, and replace them with these healthier, unsaturated fats.

Cut the fat, keep the flavor

Nothing raises your cholesterol more than saturated fat. While cholesterol in your blood can come from dietary sources of cholesterol, such as egg yolks, it mainly comes from saturated fat. Saturated fat can even worsen your insulin resistance, making it harder to control your blood sugar.

Meats and whole milk dairy products, including butter and cheese, are notorious sources, but so are coconut and palm oils often used in nondairy whipped toppings and packaged desserts. In general, the more solid a fat is at room temperature, the more saturated. Strive to limit your saturated fat to less than 7 percent of your daily calories. It may sound hard, but it's surprisingly simple.

▶ Swap low-fat dairy products for their fatty counterparts. Replace butter, lard, and margarine with spreads and oils made from corn, sunflower, and safflower oils. Use low-fat or nonfat milk instead of cream in sauces.

▶ Eat fish, legumes, bulgur, and rice for your protein instead of meat. Try using beans and tofu instead of meat in casseroles, soups, and stews.

▶ Steam, poach, broil, grill, microwave, or bake foods rather than sauté or pan-fry them. Cook meat on a rack so the fat drains off.

▶ Take advantage of healthful cookware, such as microwave ovens, vegetable steamers, pressure cookers, and nonstick pots and pans. These help foods keep their nutrients and make cooking them a little easier as well.

▶ Trim excess fat off meat. Trimming the fat off a pork chop, for example, can lower the saturated fat from 13 grams to 4 grams.

▶ Skim the fat off soups or stews. If possible, cook the broth in advance, chill, then remove the hardened layer of fat.

▶ Perk up flavors with balsamic vinegar, sun-dried tomatoes, Dijon mustard, Tabasco sauce, salsa, catsup, green chilies, or small amounts of sesame or hot chili oils.

▶ Season vegetables with herbs and spices instead of high-fat butter and sauces. Don't be afraid to experiment with new seasonings.

▶ Cut back the fat in your favorite recipes by a third, and replace the fat in baked recipes with applesauce or puréed prunes.

▶ Make your own reduced-fat dressing by using more vinegar and less oil. Use lemon juice and Italian herbs for fat-free flavor.

Saturated fat isn't your only enemy. There's an even more danger-ous one hidden in some of your favorite foods. Trans fat is a sneaky, polyunsaturated fat gone awry. During processing, manufacturers turn some of a food's unsaturated fat into saturated fat to extend its shelf life or change the taste or texture. Trans fatty acids are one of the byproducts. This unusual kind of super-fat raises your LDL cho-lesterol, may lower your HDL, and increases your risk for diabetes, heart disease, and possibly cancer. Baked goods, french fries, stick margarine, and hydrogenated vegetable oils are prime sources.

Major sources of trans fat

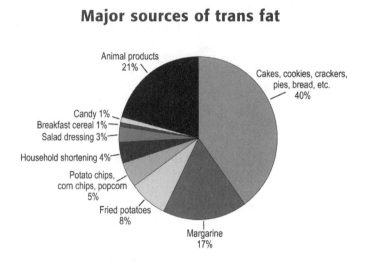

U.S. Food and Drug Administration

Avoid eating foods high in trans fat. Studies show it can raise your LDL cholesterol levels and increase your risk of coronary heart disease. The graph above shows major sources of trans fat for American adults. You can use it as a guideline or check nutrition labels on foods to find out how much trans fat they have.

Kim Severson, author of *The Trans Fat Solution: Cooking and Shopping to Eliminate the Deadliest Fat from Your Diet,* has some good suggestions on finding and avoiding this dangerous fat.

Read the label. Check the list of ingredients for partially hydrogenated vegetable oil. Hydrogenation is the process of shooting hydrogen through liquid vegetable oil. This makes it solid at room temperature and increases shelf life. If this ingredient is among the first few on the label, look for a different brand.

Avoid the obvious. Most packaged baked goods, like muffins, doughnuts, cookies, crackers, and cakes, are guaranteed to contain large amounts of trans fats. Brownie mixes, nondairy creamers, whipped dessert toppings, and processed dinners are also obvious targets. Watch out for the unexpected – certain breakfast cereals and bars, microwave popcorn, flour tortillas, processed cheese, and frozen french fries, potpies, and pizzas have hidden trans fats.

Cook more often. Because products made with trans fats stay fresher and have a better texture, they're in everything from potato chips to cereals. Learn to prepare as much of your food as possible from fresh ingredients. Shop at whole-foods markets. They often have entire lines of trans-fat-free products.

Inquire at restaurants. Fast food chains are notorious for using trans fat to fry everything. Upscale restaurants make a bigger effort to use vegetable oils. If a fried entrée catches your interest, ask your server to find out what type of oil they use for frying. If it's liquid vegetable oil, you can eat it without worrying about trans fats.

Make room for healthy foods. On the other hand, you want to make room for more soluble fiber and plant sterols and stanols, which block the absorption of cholesterol as it moves through your digestive tract. Aim for 10 to 25 daily grams of soluble fiber, which you'll find in oats, barley, beans, and fruits and vegetables. Look for margarines or other foods, like orange juice, that have been fortified with plant sterols or stanols. Just 2 grams a day helps lower cholesterol.

Get the skinny on fat substitutes

A margarine you can spread on your toast that's kind to your heart? It may sound too good to be true, but this margarine actually clobbers artery-clogging cholesterol thanks to two plant compounds called stanols and sterols. Sterols from soybeans are the power behind Take Control margarine. Stanol is the secret weapon in the canola-based Benecol margarine.

Both substances work by blocking your body's absorption of cholesterol. "Stanols and sterols bind with cholesterol found in food and with bile acids used to make cholesterol in the body," says Lona Sandon, assistant professor of clinical nutrition at The University of Texas Southwestern Medical Center at Dallas. This binding prevents cholesterol from being absorbed into the bloodstream, she says.

You're more likely to have heart disease if you have too much low-density lipoprotein (LDL) cholesterol. That's why LDL is nicknamed "bad" cholesterol. But stanol and sterol margarines can help. A review of more than 40 research studies concluded that

The low-fat trap

Because of the current war against fat, many people are trying to lose weight by removing fat from their diets. To make matters worse, they often replace these fat calories with simple carbohydrates like sugar and honey. Low-fat diet foods are notorious for adding back taste by piling on the sugar. Don't be fooled.

Even though fat is under attack, calories still count. And pound for pound, simple sugar calories stimulate the most insulin production in your body. The best way to safely control your weight and guard against diabetes is to eat a well-rounded diet, complete with foods rich in polyunsaturated fats, such as sunflower oil or safflower oil, or monounsaturated fats, such as olive oil, canola oil, avocados, and nuts.

Instead of loading up on sweets, round out your diet with foods high in complex carbohydrates like fruits and vegetables.

just 2 grams of stanols or sterols daily could help cut LDL cholesterol levels by about 10 percent. Stanol and sterol margarines are
most helpful if your cholesterol is only modestly high – around
200 to 239 mg/dL.

The National Institutes of Health (NIH) guidelines for lowering
cholesterol recommend 2 grams of plant stanols, found in
Benecol; or sterols, found in Take Control, every day. Read the
label to see how much of the spread you'll need to get the suggested amount. Eating more than 2 grams daily won't help and is
not recommended.

Although stanol and sterol margarines are generally recognized as
safe, the products haven't been around long enough for long-term
safety studies. One problem experts do know – they keep your
body from absorbing important fat-soluble nutrients, like beta
carotene and vitamin E.

"These margarines may lower carotenoid levels in the blood by 10
to 20 percent," Sandon says. But you can fix that by eating five or
more servings of vegetables daily. Make sure, she warns, you
include one food high in beta carotene such as carrots, sweet potatoes, pumpkin, tomatoes, apricots, spinach, or broccoli. Follow these
steps to make the best use of these new margarines.

▶ To get maximum mileage from your margarine, use it to replace
   fats you normally eat. Otherwise, you'll gain weight and cancel
   out the spread's benefits.

▶ Don't use these margarines to replace your medication.
   Although the spreads work well with cholesterol-lowering medicines, like statins, they're no substitute. Combine them with a
   low-fat diet or medication, however, and you might cut your
   LDL up to 20 percent.

▶ Check the labels if you plan to use the margarine for cooking or
   want zero trans-fats. "Some versions of the products are trans-fat
   free, which means they contain less than 0.5 grams of trans-fat
   per serving. The regular stanol margarines that can be used for

baking and cooking contain less than 1 gram of trans-fat per serving," says Sandon.

▸ Talk with your doctor before trying sterol or stanol margarines, especially if you take cyclosporine or similar medications.

If you don't normally eat margarine, look for the "Take Heart" line of products by Altus Foods. These include cereals, snack bars, and fruit juices – all made with plant sterols. You can cut back on bad fats in other ways, too, starting with this advice.

Get on board with DAG. Regular cooking oils, even the healthy ones, are triglyceride-based (TAG), and your body tends to store them as fat. Diacylglycerols (DAGs), like Enova, are different. Your body processes more of them in the liver and stores less as fat. New research finds replacing regular cooking oils with DAGs delays kidney failure and the need for dialysis in diabetic nephropathy, while these oils helped lower triglycerides in people with diabetes in a past study.

You can use DAGs in place of other oils in salad dressing, baking, sautéing, and frying. They're still high in fat – mostly the healthier, unsaturated kind – and still pack a whopping 120 calories per tablespoon just like regular oils, so don't overdo it. Remember that some TAGs like olive oil are good for your heart, so don't totally replace them in your diet.

Eat right with Oatrim. Meet the cholesterol-fighting fat substitute made from beta-glucan, the soluble fiber in oats. It's called Oatrim. Add it to recipes and it supplies cholesterol-busting beta-glucan, yet it has only 1 calorie per gram. Fat has 9 calories per gram. The food industry already uses Oatrim to slash fat. Supermarkets, for instance, will soon be selling a new type of low-fat milk made from cow's milk with the taste, look, and mouth-feel of whole milk, but the fat has been replaced with Oatrim. To find more products made with it, look for "hydrolyzed oat bran" in the ingredient list.

Prep for more protein

Your body can digest and use animal protein more easily than plant protein. Legumes are next easiest to digest, followed by grains and other plant sources. Cooking protein foods with moist rather than dry heat, perhaps boiled in a stew rather than fried, or soaking meat in a marinade using wine, lemon juice, or vinegar makes it easier to digest.

Bake without butter. When a baking recipe calls for butter or oil, fat-watchers often use applesauce or puréed prunes instead. A recent study found another surprising fat substitute – pawpaw purée. The pawpaw is an oblong, yellow-green fruit that grows in the eastern U.S. and Canada, and tastes a little like a mango or banana. If you mash the pulp in a blender or food processor, you end up with a healthy alternative to oil.

If you'd rather use puréed prunes, just purée about 1 1/3 cups of pitted prunes with 6 tablespoons of hot water. This should make about a cup of prune purée that will keep in the refrigerator for up to one month. Use half the recommended fat in a recipe, then add half that amount of puréed prunes. For example, if a recipe calls for a cup of oil or butter, use 1/2 cup of oil, then add 1/4 cup of prune purée. You can use this purée in cakes, muffins, cookies, and even brownies.

Find fake fats. Fat substitutes allow you to enjoy an occasional high-fat snack without worrying that your cholesterol level will skyrocket. Olestra (Olean), for example, takes potato chips off the high-danger list. It can't increase your cholesterol because your body won't digest it, and it passes through without giving you any calories from fat. But it may cause some unpleasant side effects in your intestinal tract, like cramping and diarrhea. Worse, even small amounts of olestra can deplete your body of certain vitamins and minerals that may protect against diseases like cancer.

Still, replacing a third of your normal fats and fatty snacks with those made with olestra may help you lose weight and improve your cholesterol. Giving yourself the green light to eat more junk because it's made with olestra, however, does not.

How to pick lean, mean protein

Protein is a part of every cell in your body, and no other nutrient plays as many different roles in keeping you alive and healthy. It's important for the growth and repair of your muscles, bones, skin, tendons, ligaments, hair, eyes, and other tissues. Without it, you would lack the enzymes and hormones you need for metabolism, digestion, and other important processes.

Your body needs different kinds of protein, which it pieces together from about 20 "building blocks" called amino acids. Nine of these are essential amino acids, which means you must get them from food. The others are nonessential. This doesn't mean you don't need them. You just don't have to eat them because your body can make them.

Moderate amounts of protein may help balance your blood sugar. Unlike most refined carbohydrates, protein does not cause glucose levels to spike, making it a smart choice at mealtime. Most experts advise people with diabetes to get 10 to 20 percent of their daily calories from protein, and a new Finnish study suggests poultry may be the best way to do that. Out of more than 4,000 men and women, those who made poultry part of a healthy diet had less chance of developing type 2 diabetes.

It's easiest to get protein from meat, chicken, turkey, fish, and dairy foods. Cooked meat is about 15 to 40 percent protein. Foods from animal sources provide complete protein, which means they contain all the essential amino acids. Next to meat, legumes – beans, peas, and peanuts – have the most protein. But they are called incomplete proteins because they lack some essential amino acids. You can get complete protein if you combine legumes with a serving of grains, seeds, nuts, or vegetables. Eat at least two of any of these plant foods, with or without beans, and you get complete protein.

You don't have to eat these foods in the same dish, or even in the same meal. But many cultures have created combinations that work well – like corn and beans in Mexico, or rice and split peas in India. Many Americans enjoy legumes and grains in a peanut butter sandwich.

You only need about 10 to 15 percent of your total calories from protein. Chances are, you eat a lot more than that – probably too much, especially from meat sources. The typical Western diet includes about 100 grams of protein, while 50 grams is closer to what your body needs. And it's easy enough to achieve. A five-ounce portion of lean meat, chicken, or fish contains about 35 grams of protein. Two cups of skim milk have 16 grams of protein, and one cup of nonfat yogurt has 12 grams.

Moderate amounts of protein may benefit your blood sugar health, but experts warn against extreme high-protein diets for people with diabetes. Such a diet may affect how well your kidneys work and impact long-term heart health, both special dangers for people with diabetes. Plus, high-protein sources like meat are often high in fat, too. If you don't watch the fat content, you risk weight gain, heart disease, and worsening diabetes. Pick the best protein and chuck the fat with lean choices like these.

▸ Focus on fish and skinless turkey and chicken. They're lower in fat than beef and pork. Legumes and tofu (soybean curd) offer other low-fat protein choices.

▸ Choose beef cuts with "loin" or "round" in the name.

▸ Pick "choice" instead of "prime," and choose cuts graded "USDA Select."

▶ When buying pork, pick cuts with the word "loin" or "leg" in the name.

▶ Trim away excess fat once you've chosen your meat carefully.

▶ Give up frying your food. Bake, broil, roast, or microwave it instead.

▶ Eat only low-fat or fat-free dairy products. You'll get the same nutrients, including dairy protein, without the saturated fat.

Take a fresh look at filling your plate

You may have learned to ignore wild claims about fad diets, but sometimes it's hard to understand advice from reliable sources. The U.S. Department of Agriculture (USDA) food pyramid, for example, can be confusing, especially if you forget it's three-dimensional – with height, width, and depth. The base of the pyramid represents a lot more rice, bread, cereal, and pasta than you might realize if you view it as a triangle having only height and width.

And keeping up with RDAs and DRIs, food groups, and serving sizes is enough to make you throw up your hands – or reach for a bag of potato chips. Here's how to simplify your meals and your life.

Picture your plate. To show you at a glance how a healthy arrangement of food actually looks on your plate, nutritionists at the American Institute for Cancer Research (AICR) created an eating plan called The New American Plate.

Vegetables, fruits, whole grains, and beans cover two-thirds or more of this plate. That's because a diet based mostly on plant foods lowers your risk of many diseases. Be sure you include hearty helpings of different vegetables and fruits. Don't fill all that space with pasta and whole-grain bread.

Meat, fish, poultry, or low-fat dairy foods cover no more than one-third of The New American Plate. Stick to a recommended serving of no more than 3 ounces of meat by mixing it with vegetables, grains, and beans in a stir-fry, stew, or casserole.

Size up a simple serving. What you think you eat and what you really eat may be quite different. A USDA survey compared what people said they ate with what they really ate. Most underestimated the amounts of some foods and overestimated others.

This confusion probably occurs because people don't understand how much food a serving really is. To make it clearer, the AICR suggests you measure out standard servings of foods and put them into your usual bowl or plate. One cup is the standard serving of most cereals, for example. You may be surprised at how it looks in your bowl. What you considered one serving may be closer to two.

Pay attention to portion sizes when you eat out, too. Many restaurants have switched from the traditional 10-inch to 12-inch plate, but you don't have to load it up. Here's another healthy idea – turn down the larger amounts in those fast-food deals like "value meals" and "super-sizing." Everybody likes saving a buck, but bad health is not a bargain.

Stay slim with a lifetime eating plan. The New American Plate was not designed to be a weight-loss diet. "But it does show people how to enjoy all foods in sensible portions," says Melanie Polk, AICR Director for Nutrition Education. "Thus, it promotes a healthy weight as one aspect of an overall healthy lifestyle."

If you forget fad diets and stick to this plan, Polk believes, you won't have to worry about obesity. "All the fad diets with their high-protein, low-sugar, low-carbohydrate directives," she says, "have confused people about some basic principles."

Ignore any diet that encourages you to cut back on the fruits and vegetables that help prevent chronic disease. You don't want to put your long-term health at risk for short-term weight loss.

In addition to selecting healthy foods, pay attention to the calories you take in. "Once you suit your portions to your needs," says Polk, "you will find it easier to maintain a healthy weight for life."

Small changes can make a big difference. "Choosing the regular burger instead of the quarter-pound burger, Polk points out, "saves 160 calories."

If you'd like a free copy of The New American Plate brochure, call 800-843-8114. More information is available on the AICR Web site at *www.aicr.org.*

Smelly herb outsmarts illness

Garlic has been appreciated for thousands of years for its healing powers as well as its flavor. The ancient Egyptian and Chinese cultures used the fragrant bulb as medicine. Slaves building the pyramids ate garlic to keep up their strength. Aristotle praised its medicinal powers. Roman warriors ate it to give them courage in battle. Even the Bible mentions garlic. During their long trek through the desert after leaving Egypt, the Israelites said garlic was one of the foods they missed.

Not only is garlic just as popular today, but scientific research says eating garlic may indeed provide health benefits. In fact, garlic may protect you from just about everything from the common cold to diabetes and cancer. It might even help you live longer.

So what is it about garlic that makes it so special? Crush garlic and it produces a powerful, penicillin-like compound called allicin. Allicin, in turn, breaks down to create several sulfur compounds plus a substance called ajoene. These compounds give garlic its distinctive smell. In addition, garlic is chock-full of antioxidants that protect you from damaging free radicals and is a good source of selenium, an important trace element.

Sow garlic and reap the rewards

Eating garlic can do wonders for your health. So can gardening. Why not combine the two? In fall, when temperatures are cool, plant garlic cloves 4 to 8 inches apart in fertile, slightly moist, well-drained soil.

Plant more than you need and keep a close eye on the leaves. When the lower leaves turn brown or yellow, harvest time is near. Harvest it before the temperature gets too warm. Usually that means May in the South and July in the North. Eight to 10 days before harvest, stop watering and let the soil dry thoroughly before digging up the bulbs.

To find out whether the time is right, dig up one or two whole plants — roots, shoots, and all. Cut open the bulb. If the cloves inside have separated, start harvesting your other garlic plants, too.

Along with its mythological warding off of vampires, garlic may scare off diabetes and the complications that come with it. This odiferous herb is said to lower blood sugar, blood pressure, triglycerides, and "bad" LDL cholesterol. It also may improve circulation, keep your blood platelets from clumping together, and help prevent hardening of the arteries, although recent studies have not supported those claims. The sulfur-containing compounds that make garlic so smelly may be responsible for any possible benefits.

Just a clove of garlic (about 4 grams) a day will do it — but check with your doctor first if you're taking warfarin or other blood-thinning medications. Start working fresh garlic into two or three recipes a week. Buy firm bulbs with white, papery skin, and store them in a cool, dry place.

Get to the 'heart' of diabetes prevention

Most people with diabetes die from some form of heart disease. In fact, the American Heart Association says the relationship between these two conditions is so important, they believe diabetes IS a cardiovascular disease.

If you have diabetes, you are twice as likely to have high blood pressure as someone who doesn't. The extra pressure means your heart must work extra hard to pump blood through your body, and that strain can lead to heart disease. In fact, high blood pressure may cause up to 75 percent of all cardiovascular disease in people with diabetes. Even though you can't see the damage, years of high blood pressure can injure your arteries, setting you up for a heart attack later.

The American Diabetes Association recommends keeping your blood pressure below 130/85. Start by watching the sodium in your diet. It's a major mineral in salt, and a major enemy to your heart. Sodium lends a hand in regulating your body fluids and blood pressure, and helps muscles and nerves work properly. Your body only needs a tiny bit − about 600 milligrams (mg) − to regulate fluids and control blood pressure, among other jobs. Most people, however, eat more than 3,000 mg of sodium each day.

Limiting your sodium to less than 2,400 mg a day could put a lid on high blood pressure. People who are salt-sensitive and already have high blood pressure could especially benefit from eating less salt. Your bones will thank you, too. Your kidneys flush out extra sodium in your urine. Unfortunately, a lot of other important minerals, like calcium, get flushed out as well. The more sodium you eat, the more calcium you lose. The more calcium you lose, the greater your bone loss and risk for osteoporosis.

Naturally, the best way to cut back sodium is to eat less salt and salty foods, but simply hiding the saltshaker is not enough. Here's where most people get their sodium.

Grow a longer life

Working in your garden is good for your heart. And the antioxidant herbs you grow there — oregano, dill, rosemary, and parsley — can help your heart by fighting high cholesterol and lowering blood pressure. If you want to fight clogged arteries, grow garlic. And to help cut back on salt, which could contribute to high blood pressure, grow chives, sage, basil, and other flavorful herbs to spice up your food.

Gardening also helps your heart by reducing stress. And when the work is done, relax even more with the scent of lavender blossoms while you sip a soothing cup of homegrown chamomile tea.

▶ 10 percent from the natural salt content of foods

▶ 15 percent from salt added at the table or during cooking

▶ 75 percent from salt added to foods during processing and manufacturing

As you can see, while some foods naturally contain small amounts of sodium, most of it is added during cooking or processing to boost flavor.

Find creative salt substitutes. A great way to reduce salt is to find high-flavor replacements. Red wine vinegar or balsamic vinegar can make tempting and tasty salt substitutes. So can spices, herbs, lemon juice, or lime juice. Garlic and onions improve almost any meal. What's more, these choices can lower the fat in your diet to help you lose weight. Try using these seasonings in place of cream sauces, butter, gravies, mayonnaise, or salad dressings. You'll still get the flavor, but without so much fat and salt.

Load up on fruits and veggies. In their natural, fresh form, they're low in sodium and packed with potassium, a mineral that may help reduce blood pressure. Take corn, for example. A cup of cooked fresh corn has 226 mg of potassium and 8 mg of sodium, the main ingredient in salt. That's a healthy ratio in anyone's diet. But what if you ate a cup of corn flakes instead? After all the processing, the corn is left with only 20 mg of potassium and a whopping 228 mg of sodium. Obviously, you're better off with the fresh food.

Rethink your eating habits. You may be surprised to learn that some salty foods are actually better choices than foods that don't taste salty. Salted peanuts, for example, contain less sodium than instant chocolate pudding. But you notice the salt more because it directly touches your taste buds. Remember that when it comes to seasoning your food during cooking. A light sprinkling of salt at the table may be healthier and more satisfying than loading it on beforehand.

Spot hidden sources. Salt can pop up in some surprising places, like your medication. Among over-the-counter drugs, antacids, laxatives, anti-inflammatory drugs, and cold medicines may contain large amounts of sodium. To find out how much sodium is hiding in the medication you take, read the labels on over-the-counter drugs. And ask your pharmacist to check the package inserts that come with prescription drugs.

Another unexpected source, baking soda, might seem like the perfect answer to your heartburn problem, but one-half teaspoon of Arm & Hammer Baking Soda contains a whopping 616 mg of sodium.

Get back to nature. Processed foods, such as frozen dinners, instant rice and pasta mixes, salad dressings, and canned soups and broths contribute the most salt in your diet. Nearly a third of the sodium you eat likely comes from store-bought baked goods and cereal. Foods made from milk also tend to be high in salt. Even worse, most of the minerals that help lower blood pressure are lost when fresh foods are processed.

Try to eat fresh, unsalted, or low-sodium foods whenever you can. Read labels. Products low in sodium often advertise that fact. Check the Nutrition Facts label, too, and look for foods with less than 5 percent − about 120 mg − of your maximum daily sodium allowance. You can cut the sodium in canned vegetables and meats up to 40 percent just by rinsing them with water before you eat them.

Go easy on the sides. Pickled foods, ketchup, mustard, horseradish, and barbecue sauces can carry lots of sodium. Treat even low-sodium versions of soy and teriyaki sauces like salt, and use them sparingly.

Mind your meats. Most processed meats like bologna and hot dogs are pumped full of sodium to keep them moist and fresh. Buy fresh or frozen fish, poultry, and meat, instead. These tend to have less salt than their canned and processed counterparts. The exceptions are cured meats like bacon and ham, which are usually loaded with sodium.

Eat at home. Most restaurants add salt and salt-rich sauces for flavor. Try to eat most of your meals at home. When you prepare your own food using fresh fruits, vegetables, and meat, you can control how much salt you get. Eat less salt at other meals if you're planning a fast-food run. Avoid fried dishes, mayonnaise, and other sauces, and downsize − don't "supersize."

Learn to bake with less sodium. You can cut the salt in most baked recipes in half. Yeast breads require around one-fourth teaspoon of salt per cup of flour. Use liquid vegetable oils in recipes instead of salted butter. Beware of baking powder as well − one teaspoon could pack almost 500 milligrams of sodium. Most cake recipes need only a teaspoon of baking powder per cup of flour; muffins, biscuits, and waffles take a minimum of one and one-fourth teaspoons per cup of flour.

Don't be fooled by food labels

Knowing what food-label terms mean will help you make the healthiest shopping decisions. Keep in mind that a food's serving size may be much smaller or larger than what you consider a single serving. For instance, pretzels actually contain 1 or 2 grams of fat per cup but are considered fat-free because of the small serving size used. Remember this secret when reading food labels. All the numbers given on the following pages are per-serving.

Sugar free	Less than 0.5 grams (g) of sugar
Calorie free	Less than five calories
Sodium free	Less than 5 milligrams (mg) of sodium
Fat free	Less than 0.5 g of fat
Saturated or trans fat free	Less than 0.5 g of saturated fat and 0.5 g of trans fat
Cholesterol free	No more than 2 mg of cholesterol and 2 g of saturated and trans fats combined
Low sugar	This term is not regulated, so it may not mean what you expect. Compare several brands of the same food and choose the one with the least sugar.
Low calorie	No more than 40 calories
Low sodium	No more than 140 mg of sodium
Very low sodium	No more than 35 mg of sodium
Low fat	No more than 3 grams of fat
Low cholesterol	No more than 20 mg of cholesterol and 2 g of saturated fat
Less saturated fat	Less than 25 percent of the total saturated and trans fats of the regular version

Reduced saturated fat	At least 25 percent less saturated fat (must be at least 1 g less per serving) than the regular version
Less or reduced cholesterol	At least 25 percent less cholesterol than the regular version and no more than 2 g of saturated fat
Reduced sodium, reduced calorie	At least 25 percent less sodium or calories than the regular version
Good source of calcium	At least 100 milligrams (mg) of calcium
Good source of fiber	Between 2.5 g and 4.9 g of fiber
Good source of (any nutrient)	10 to 19 percent of the recommended daily value (DV) for that nutrient
High fiber	At least 5 g of fiber. "High fiber" foods must be low-fat or include the amount of total fat next to the high-fiber claim.
High in, rich in, or excellent source of (any nutrient)	20 percent or more of the DV for that nutrient
Light or lite	One-third fewer calories or half the fat of the regular version; or half the sodium of a low-calorie, low-fat food. May also refer to the texture or color of the product, as in "light brown sugar."
Extra lean	Less than 5 g of fat, 2 g of saturated and trans fat combined, and 95 mg of cholesterol.
Lean	Less than 10 g of fat, 4 g of saturated and trans fat combined, and 95 mg of cholesterol per serving of fish, poultry, or meat

Nutty way to nix diabetes

Researchers with the Nurses' Health Study recently looked at the relationship between nuts and diabetes risk, and they liked what they saw. Women in the study who ate an ounce of nuts – about a handful – at least five times a week had a 27-percent less chance of developing type 2 diabetes, compared with women who almost never ate them. Other studies have shown that eating nuts at least five times a week can slash your risk of heart attack in half.

"We were not really surprised by our findings," says Rui Jiang, an author of the diabetes study. "Nuts contain lots of fat, but most fats in nuts are mono- and polyunsaturated fats, which are good for insulin sensitivity and serum cholesterol. Nuts are also rich in antioxidant vitamins, minerals, plant protein, and dietary fiber."

They're also cholesterol-free, and most are low in the saturated fats that send cholesterol skyward. In addition, many nuts serve up arginine, an amino acid your body uses to fight plaque buildup in your arteries, while the folic acid in nuts keeps too much homocysteine from piling up in your blood and harming arteries. What's more, their soluble fiber may cut LDL cholesterol, and many nuts provide heart-healthy minerals like copper and magnesium.

What more can you ask for? Be a health nut. Sprinkle them in salads or cereals, add them to baked goods, or just grab a handful for a healthy snack. Try these nuts on for size – and variety.

Wise up to walnuts. A great source of good, polyunsaturated omega-3 fats, walnuts are proven to lower cholesterol and are loaded with the antioxidant vitamin E. Scientists think omega-3s may pitch in to avert the irregular heartbeat that can cause "sudden death" – death within an hour of a heart attack.

The Food and Drug Administration (FDA) recently approved a health claim for walnuts saying "supportive but not conclusive research" shows that eating 1.5 ounces of walnuts daily may reduce heart disease risk – but only if the nuts don't boost calorie intake and are part of a low-cholesterol, low-saturated-fat diet. The FDA is considering a similarly worded claim for most other nuts.

Pick pecans. These nuts, rich in heart-healthy monounsaturated fat (MUFA), helped reduce total cholesterol by 6.7 percent and LDL cholesterol by 10.4 percent, according to research findings. Their high fat content can also invite rancidity. Store shelled pecans in the refrigerator for up to three months or the freezer for up to six months.

Toast almonds. Popping almonds may help ditch diabetes, thanks to their stores of MUFAs, protein, and fiber. The American Diabetes Association (ADA) says MUFAs could help manage your insulin and blood sugar levels, lower cholesterol, and fight diabetes-related heart disease. In fact, these special fatty acids make up a big part of the ADA's eating plan.

A review of nut research found that nut eaters don't have a higher body mass index than folks who don't eat nuts – as long as the nuts replace another high-calorie food in their diet. Jiang agrees. "To avoid increase in caloric intake," she advises, "people should not simply add nuts on the top of the diet. Instead, people should substitute nuts for less-healthy foods such as refined carbohydrates, like white bread and red meats." Otherwise, you and your waistline are in for an unpleasant surprise.

Avoid nuts coated with candy, sugar, honey, or salt. If you're salt-sensitive, check the label for sodium content. Nuts are a common cause of food allergies. Call for emergency help if you experience any of these symptoms within an hour of eating nuts – skin rash, scratchy or swollen throat, stuffy or runny nose, sneezing, difficulty breathing, stomach upset, vomiting, diarrhea, or bloating.

Nuts	Nuts per 1-ounce serving	Calories	Protein (grams)	Fat (grams)				Omega-6 fatty acids (grams)	Omega-3 fatty acids (grams)	Vitamin E or alpha-tocopherol (milligrams)
				Total	Sat	Mono	Poly			
Almonds	24 nuts	160	6	14	1	9	3	3	0	7.3
Brazils	6-8 nuts	190	4	19	5	7	7	6.8	0.02	1.6
Cashews (dry roasted)	18 nuts	160	4	13	3	8	2	2.2	0.05	0.3
Hazelnuts	20 nuts	180	4	17	1.5	13	2	2.2	0.02	4.3
Macadamias (dry roasted)	10-12 nuts	200	2	22	3	17	0.5	0.4	0.06	0.2
Peanuts	28 nuts	170	7	14	2	7	5	4.4	0	2
Pecans	20 halves	200	3	20	2	12	6	5.9	0.28	0.4
Pine nuts (pignolias)	157	190	4	20	2	6	10	9.4	0.05	2.6
Pistachios (dry roasted)	49 nuts	160	6	13	1.5	7	4	3.9	0.07	0.6
Walnuts	14 halves	190	4	18	1.5	2.5	13	10.8	2.6	0.2

Red Bush tea: a powerful ally

Who would have thought drinking a hot, soothing beverage every day could prevent diabetic vision loss? Sound too good to be true? Evidence links Red Bush tea with amazing protective powers.

Tea is still a popular beverage after thousands of years, and it's no wonder when you consider all its benefits. History credits the Chinese with discovering this delicious drink in 2737 B.C. by a fortunate accident. Emperor Shen-Nung was boiling water on his terrace when leaves from a nearby bush blew over and fell into the water. He tried it and thought it tasted great. Before long, people all over China and the rest of East Asia were making tea. The Dutch and British started importing tea during the 17th century, but they preferred black tea.

Now another kind, Red Bush tea, is making waves. Known in its native South Africa as "Rooibos" (ROY-boss), Dutch for "red bush," it comes from the needle-shaped leaves of the *Aspalathus linearis* bush.

True to its name, it makes a fragrant cup of reddish brown tea that's caffeine-free. Best of all, it's rich in antioxidant compounds called catechins. These might prevent vision loss from diabetic retinopathy and cataracts by keeping a lid on the amount of free radicals in your blood

Make the best of Red Bush tea

Red Bush tea from South Africa may be more potent than the varieties grown in other African countries. You can get it loose or in tea bags. If you buy it loose, look for leaves with an even color and delicate, rather than strong, aroma. Steep it for 5 to 10 minutes. The longer it steeps and the hotter the water, the more antioxidants you get.

and eye lenses. Take the time to kick back and relax with a cup of Red Bush tea. You'll be doing your body a favor.

Oats even out sugar spikes

You've heard the expression "healthy as a horse." And you probably know horses often eat oats. Coincidence? Doubtful. You don't have to strap on a feedbag, but you might want to gallop to the grocery store for some of this healthy grain. The outer husk of the oat grain contains tons of beta-glucan, a sticky form of soluble fiber that slows down your food as it travels through your stomach and small intestine.

This slows your absorption of carbohydrates, so your blood doesn't get flooded with glucose all at once and create an immediate and urgent demand for insulin. That's good news for people with diabetes, who need to keep tight control of blood sugar levels. Experts say doubling, even tripling, the amount of soluble fiber in your diet can improve glycemic control. Oats can help you do that. Research has shown adding oat bran to meals lowers after-meal spikes in glucose and insulin better than wheat bran in both healthy people and those with type 2 diabetes.

The form of oat you eat also plays a part – the less processed the grain, the better. Steel-cut oats undergo the least processing. Unfortunately, most oats you buy in the store are some form of oat groats, which are processed by removing the outer layer, toasting, and cleaning the oat. Rolled oats, or old-fashioned oats, are simply oat groats that have been steamed and flattened. Other varieties include Scotch oats and Irish oatmeal, which have been cut but not rolled. You can also buy oat bran or oat flour. If you can't find these products in your supermarket, try a health food store.

Oats also serve up a delicious boost of protein and a variety of key minerals like potassium, magnesium, phosphorous, manganese, copper, and zinc. Aside from beating diabetes, eating a healthy portion of oats each day can help you lower your cholesterol, prevent colon cancer, and cure constipation. When it comes to fighting disease, all it takes is some oats and old-fashioned horse sense.

Cut your cholesterol. Adding just one serving of oats to your diet should help if you have high cholesterol. By slowing down the digestion of food, oats give good, high-density lipoprotein (HDL) more time to pick up cholesterol and whisk it to the liver and out of the body. It also gives bad, low-density lipoprotein (LDL) less chance to move cholesterol to your artery walls, where it can build up and cause problems.

Some studies have reported that oats slashed total cholesterol by as much as 26 percent and LDL cholesterol by 24 percent, but most experts are more cautious. Researchers concluded that 3 grams of beta-glucan could slightly lower cholesterol. Since even a modest reduction leads to a lower risk of heart disease, this is big news. Even the Food and Drug Administration (FDA) has endorsed oat products for their cholesterol-lowering ability. If you have high cholesterol, you'll see a more dramatic dip than if your cholesterol levels are normal or low.

Cancel out colon cancer. Beta-glucan rides to the rescue once again. Although it slows food as it passes through your stomach and small intestine, it speeds food through your large intestine, which lowers your risk of colon cancer. It may also react with tiny organisms there to form compounds that protect the colon wall and tame cancer-causing substances.

Give yourself an 'egg' up

Egg white is high in protein, riboflavin, and lysine, and it does almost everything whole eggs do — but without the tiniest hint of fat or cholesterol.

Kick constipation. The fiber in oats also keeps your digestive system running smoothly and prevents constipation. Remember, fiber acts as a natural laxative. It helps your colon form stools soft enough to pass quickly and easily through your system. Just make sure to drink plenty of water when you add more fiber to your diet.

Get the most from your oats with this key advice.

▶ Start your day with a bowl of oatmeal or oat bran cereal. You can also sprinkle oat bran on your cereal or baked goods.

▶ Cook oat groats as a side dish, like rice, or use them in salads or stuffings.

▶ Take your time. While instant oatmeal may be quicker than cooking old-fashioned oats, remember it also contains added sugar and salt.

▶ Think ahead. Because it's less processed, steel-cut oatmeal takes longer to cook. Soak the oats overnight to shorten the cooking time.

▶ Cook your oatmeal with fat-free milk for extra nutrition and diabetes-prevention.

▶ Oats makes a great binder in recipes. Add one-fourth cup of oats to pancake batter or to meat loaves and patties. You can add oat bran to almost any recipe for bread, rolls, and biscuits, too.

▶ Change it up. If you get tired of oats, consider barley, another good source of beta-glucan.

Act fast to boost low blood sugar

Sudden grouchiness, hunger, or tiredness might not just be a passing mood. If you have diabetes, it could be a sign of hypoglycemia or low blood sugar. Hypoglycemia occurs when your blood sugar dips too low. Other symptoms include weakness, confusion, sweating, headache, shakiness, or even coma and seizures.

If you experience mild symptoms of hypoglycemia, take action quickly by following these steps to recovery from the National Institutes of Health. For severe hypoglycemic emergencies, you'll need special treatment.

Check your blood sugar level. A reading of 70 or lower means you are hypoglycemic. To raise your blood sugar back to a safe level, try one of these fast-acting remedies.

▶ half a cup of fruit juice or regular (not diet) soda

▶ a piece of fruit or small box of raisins

▶ five or six pieces of hard candy

▶ one to two teaspoons of sugar or honey

▶ two to three store-bought glucose tablets

Carry one of these quick fixes with you at all times. If you take insulin, keep a glucagon kit with you, too. It can quickly raise your blood glucose level.

Wait 15 minutes. Then check your blood sugar again to make sure it's no longer too low.

Make sure a meal is on the horizon. Once your blood sugar level is stable, plan to eat a meal within the next hour. If you can't, snack on one of the following:

▶ crackers, peanut butter, or cheese crackers

▶ half a sandwich

▶ a serving of milk or yogurt

Prevent future incidents. Don't gamble with your blood sugar level. Managing it is a matter of discipline and good sense. So eat regular meals and avoid alcohol. Take your medication as prescribed. Check your blood sugar often. And, last but not least, exercise with care.

Make the healthy switch to olive oil

It's not some new miracle cure. Olive oil has been prized in cooking and healing for thousands of years. The Cretes grew rich from exporting olive oil as far back as 2475 B.C., and both the Bible and Greek mythology refer to it. Now exported mainly from France, Spain, Italy, and Greece, you can find it in any supermarket.

This flavorful oil fights diabetes, heart disease, and rheumatoid arthritis plus works wonders for aging skin. Made by pressing ripe olives, olive oil is 77 percent monounsaturated fat (MUFA), the good kind that helps rather than hurts your body. Thanks to MUFAs, this tasty oil may reduce your risk of type 2 diabetes by lowering your blood sugar and cutting the amount of LDL, total cholesterol, and triglycerides (fats) in your blood.

It's also rich in vitamin E, has several cancer-resisting compounds, and may help prevent your blood from clotting, which lowers your blood pressure and risk of stroke. What olive oil doesn't have is cholesterol or salt. And it has very little saturated fat that can raise cholesterol.

People are finally catching on to this liquid gold. A record number of home cooks are using olive oil instead of vegetable oils high in saturated fat. In fact, the North American Olive Oil Association says 34 percent of all homes use olive oil, and recent sales are at all-time highs. If you want to join the rank of smart cooks, add olive oil to your list of must-have ingredients. Don't worry if you feel lost when you see all the varieties on the supermarket shelf. By focusing on three main types, you'll have an easier choice.

Extra virgin. The name refers to its purity. The ripe olives are picked and sent to the mill the same day. First, they are crushed by giant wheels. Then the mash moves to the press, which squeezes out the oil. Since this first round of processing uses no heat or chemicals, the label on the bottle will say "first cold pressed."

It has a strong, robust, fruity flavor, and the most full-bodied taste and aroma of any olive oil. And because it's less refined, it has the most of what makes olive oil good for you. Buy the darkest color to get the most phytonutrients, and drizzle it over salad or vegetables.

Virgin. This olive oil goes through more processing, so it's not quite as good for you. Its milder flavor and hint of fruitiness, however, make it a nice, all-purpose cooking oil.

Extra light. The name refers to the color and taste, not the calorie- or fat-content. It's not as healthy as extra virgin olive oil, but it makes a good replacement for vegetable oil in recipes.

Olive oil's strong flavor means you won't need much, and its monounsaturated fats help fill you up. But don't just add it to your regular diet. It has 120 calories per tablespoon. Use it to replace other fats for an equal but healthier exchange. A few more tips can help you maximize this new tool.

▶ Try substituting olive oil for butter, margarine, or other vegetable oils when you cook. By pouring out some olive oil, you'll be pouring on the health benefits.

▶ For the best flavor, use olive oil soon after opening. It has a shelf life of about two years. Be sure to check the expiration date before buying, or buy it from a store with a quick turnover.

▶ Store your "liquid gold" in a tightly capped container in a cool, dark place. It does not need to be refrigerated.

▶ Don't start eating high-fat meals thinking olive oil will save the day. Just continue to eat sensibly, and use it in place of other fats whenever possible.

Unusual vegetable gets your liver in gear

The first time you eat an artichoke, you may be a little intimidated. After all, it looks rather strange. Fortunately, beauty is only skin-deep. Hiding inside is a nutritious, nutty-flavored treat.

One medium artichoke has about 60 calories. It's a good source of potassium, magnesium, and vitamin C, which are important for heart health. Best of all, this nutty vegetable may help regulate diabetes.

Stabilizes blood sugar. Your liver is busier than you might think. It stores extra glucose (sugar) in the form of glycogen and turns it back into glucose whenever blood supplies get too low. This is a great system in a perfectly working body. But some people have livers cranking out glucose their blood doesn't need. This overproduction can lead to diabetes and other health problems.

In animal studies, researchers found that substances in artichokes kept livers from making too much glucose. More studies need to be done, but scientists think artichokes might someday be useful to people with type 2 diabetes. You can get a jump on this exciting future by making artichokes a regular part of your menu.

Chokes off heart disease. One of your liver's main functions is to produce bile, which breaks down fats and cholesterol in the food you eat. But a liver that doesn't produce enough bile lets too much cholesterol get by – kind of like the *I Love Lucy* episode where the chocolate assembly line starts moving too fast for her to keep up. People with liver problems can have high cholesterol even if they eat a low-fat diet.

That's where artichokes come in. Because they can help you make more bile, you may be able to lower your cholesterol by eating them. A study in Germany showed that taking artichoke extract for six weeks caused LDL cholesterol, the bad kind, to fall by more than 22 percent. As a bonus, artichokes may also block some new cholesterol from forming in your liver.

Steps up digestion. Bile is necessary for good digestion. If your liver doesn't produce enough, you can't digest your food properly. If you feel sick to your stomach, overly full, and have abdominal pain after eating a normal-sized meal, you may suffer from dyspepsia — a fancy name for poor digestion.

Several scientific studies showed dramatic improvements in people with dyspepsia after being treated with artichoke extracts. You can also get help for your indigestion the way the ancient Romans did — by eating a delicious artichoke with your dinner.

Cooking artichokes is easy. Steam or boil them until tender, about 30 minutes. If you're in a hurry, cook them in your microwave. First, rinse them with water to add moisture. Then wrap each one in microwaveable plastic wrap. For four artichokes, microwave on high for 10 to 15 minutes or until the meaty part at the base of the artichoke is tender.

4 steps to eating an artichoke

There's no mystery about it — just a little finesse. Try this guide for enjoying cooked artichokes.

▶ Pluck off a petal.
▶ Hold the pointed end between your fingers and place it in your mouth.
▶ Gently scrape the petal between your teeth to remove the flavorful tasty pulp.
▶ When you reach the heart, scrape off the soft fuzz with a spoon. Then dig in and enjoy every bite.

Eat to beat high blood pressure

Monitoring your blood pressure is important, especially as you get older. The seventh annual report of the National Committee on Prevention, Detection, Evaluation, and Treatment of High Blood Pressure makes it plain:

▶ Once you reach 50 years of age and starting with a blood pressure level of 115/75 mmHg, the risk of heart disease doubles with each little increase of 20/10 mmHg.

▶ Higher than normal blood pressure is the number one attributable risk factor for death around the world.

▶ Regardless of the medication you take, high blood pressure can only be controlled if you are motivated to stay on your blood-pressure reduction plan.

These are great reasons for giving the DASH diet plan (short for Dietary Approaches to Stop Hypertension) a shot. The fact is, DASH will dramatically lower blood pressure — without additional risky drugs.

It's as simple as these natural steps, which involve eating less of some things and more of others:

▶ limit salt, trim fat, reduce red meat, and settle for fewer sweets and sweet drinks.

▶ eat more fruit, vegetables, whole grains, low-fat dairy products, poultry, and lean fish.

In short, it's a plan you can live with and enjoy.

Hear it from someone who knows. Nutritionist Mary Beth Horrell, with the Diabetes and Health Education Center at Asheville, North Carolina's Mission Hospital, can vouch for the healthfulness of the DASH diet. Her hospital's high blood pressure program has used DASH for years.

When the DASH plan was first implemented, Horrell says, it emphasized limiting fats and sweets and eating well-rounded, nutritious meals. Those who used it saw their blood pressure drop. Then DASH research began to focus on sodium, and blood pressure numbers fell even further. "The final conclusion," says Horrell, "was that both approaches are effective independently, but when combined they have the most beneficial results."

DASH zeroes in on sodium – the main ingredient in salt. "We only need 500 to 1,000 milligrams each day, so most people consume far more than they need," explains Horrell. "It's responsible for maintaining fluid balance. I tell my patients that sodium acts like

Plan your daily DASH

Here's a quick look at what you'll be eating if you take the DASH challenge.

Food group	Daily servings
grains and grain products	7-8
vegetables	4-5
fruits	4-5
dairy (low-fat or fat free)	2-3
fats and oils	2-3
meats, poultry, and fish	2 or less
nuts, seeds, and dry beans	4-5 per week
sweets	5 per week

a sponge and holds on to water. But too much sodium or water in the body causes imbalances.

"Sodium also regulates muscle contractions," she continues, "and, since our heart is a muscle, it can affect how the heart pumps. Our blood pressure is a measure of our heart beating and relaxing."

But reducing sodium isn't merely a matter of throwing the salt shaker away, Horrell says. "DASH is inherently lower in sodium because it emphasizes fresh fruits and vegetables, which have very little sodium."

Horrell believes the DASH plan is here to stay — it works and focuses on moderation. "It doesn't eliminate any food groups. It includes foods that anybody has access to. It's satisfying nutritionally. And people who use it aren't hungry. There aren't any dangers associated with DASH that I'm aware of. DASH makes sense to me."

Get the proof from research. Three major studies — DASH, DASH-Sodium, and PREMIER — all support the blood-pressure benefits of the DASH plan. These studies have proven that a diet rich in fruits, vegetables, whole grains, and low-fat dairy products and low in fat, refined carbohydrates, and sodium reduces blood pressure. What's especially exciting is the fact that DASH can lower blood pressure as much as any single blood-pressure medication can — 10, 14, even 16 points or more.

These large randomized studies also settled some long-standing debates over whether certain nutrients — like calcium, potassium, and magnesium — were blood-pressure-reducing kingpins. When they were provided in supplement form, they didn't make much difference. But when eaten in the foods of the DASH plan, the blood pressure dropped. In other words, those nutrients work best when they come from natural foods, such as those you eat in the DASH plan.

Start healing your heart. DASH is more than a diet. It's part of a lifestyle that can better your life. Your health is important, but nobody wants a "grit-your-teeth-I-can't-wait-till-this-is-over" regimen. Coupled with keeping a healthy weight, exercising regularly, and quitting smoking, DASH will help you enjoy a healthy drop in your blood pressure and cholesterol, less fatigue, and a decreased risk of heart disease and osteoporosis.

For a free copy of *Facts about the DASH Eating Plan* — including a sample week of DASH meals — visit the Web site *http://emall.nhlbihin.net.* This advice can maximize the effects of your DASH diet.

▶ Beware of sodium. "Sodium hides in everything," warns Horrell. "Salt has about 2,400 milligrams in a single teaspoon. Most processed and canned foods have excessive sodium. When you eat out, it's heavily used — especially in fast foods."

▶ Adjust to more fiber. You may experience some bloating or flatulence if you're not used to eating beans, bananas, and other high-fiber foods at DASH levels, so adjust gradually.

▶ Don't substitute supplements for good food. Get your nutrients from the wholesome, nutrient-rich DASH diet. "Magnesium, calcium, and potassium do lower blood pressure, but this combination taken in supplements doesn't show the same results," Horrell says.

Keep taking your blood-pressure medicine, and don't tamper with your dosage without first consulting your doctor. And if you slip up and overindulge, don't give up — for your blood pressure's sake.

Exotic fruit gets you back in the game

The Super Bowl generates the biggest demand for avocados all year. People eat more than 40 million pounds of avocados during the Super Bowl game. Maybe football fans are on to something.

Avocados, nicknamed "alligator pears" because of their bumpy exteriors, come in several varieties. Some have a green covering. Others are dark purple or almost black. Some are smooth, while others are bumpy. Some are small, and others weigh as much as 4 pounds. Yet, when you slice them open, they all have the same delicious, nutty-flavored flesh inside – and the same health benefits.

Crushes high cholesterol. The avocado is high in fat – 30 grams per fruit – but it's mostly monounsaturated fat. This fat helps protect good HDL cholesterol, while wiping out the bad LDL cholesterol that clogs your arteries. That means you not only lower your bad cholesterol, you also improve your ratio of good HDL to total cholesterol. An Australian study found eating half to one-and-a-half avocados a day for three weeks could lower your total cholesterol by more than 8 percent without lowering your HDL cholesterol.

But there's more than just monounsaturated fat at work. An avocado contains 10 grams of fiber, as well as a plant chemical called beta-sitosterol. These both help lower cholesterol. Throw in vitamins C and E – powerful antioxidants that prevent dangerous free radicals from reacting with the cholesterol in your blood – and it all adds up to a healthier heart.

Sidelines diabetes. Eating high-fiber foods like avocados can benefit people with type 2 diabetes in several ways. One study published in *The New England Journal of Medicine* found that a high-fiber diet (50 grams a day) lowered cholesterol, triglyceride, glucose, and insulin levels. Avocados have earned the backing of the American Diabetes Association.

Blitzes strokes. When it comes to taking on a deadly killer like stroke, who wants to play fair? Gang up on stroke with avocado's three heavyweights – potassium, magnesium, and fiber.

In the Health Professionals Follow-Up Study, which included more than 43,000 men, researchers found that the men who got the most potassium in their diet were 38 percent less likely to have a stroke as those who got the least. Results were a little lower for fiber (30 percent) and magnesium (30 percent).

Grow your own avocados

Next time you eat an avocado, save its pit. Stick three toothpicks into its side, about an inch above its flat bottom. Place the toothpicks on the rim of a cup of water so the bottom of the pit touches the water. After a few weeks, a shoot will grow out of the top and roots will grow into the water. When the roots grow into a clump as big as your fist, put potting soil in a 1-gallon container, and plant the pit.

Buy avocados that are heavy for their size and have no dark sunken spots or cracked or broken surfaces. Seal it in a plastic bag along with a ripe banana or apple to help it ripen faster, keeping the bag at room temperature. For slower ripening, store in the refrigerator. Ripe avocados should be firm but soft enough to "give way" to gentle pressure.

Not sure how to eat them? Cut the fruit lengthways around the seed and twist the halves to separate. Using a spoon, remove the seed, then scoop out the flesh and use it in one of the delicious ideas.

▶ Replace the mayonnaise in your favorite sandwich with mashed avocado for a change of pace.

▶ Mash or cube the soft fruit and mix with salsa.

▶ Float avocado cubes in a bowl of hot tomato soup.

▶ Toast a tortilla-wrapped avocado wedge.

▶ Use in place of cream cheese or butter on bagels or toast. Avocados aren't called "butterfruit" for nothing.

▶ Try it on a baked potato instead of butter or sour cream.

▶ Mash potatoes with a peeled and seeded avocado.

▶ Crown crackers with chunks of it.

▶ Fill egg white halves with guacamole for a new twist on deviled eggs.

▶ Toss some fresh slices in your tossed salads.

▶ Dice them up and drop them into an omelette.

When exposed to air, an avocado discolors quickly, so use it as soon as possible. Squeezing lemon or lime juice on the cut flesh will help prevent discoloration. To keep dips containing avocado from turning brown, place the avocado pit in them. Remove before serving. You can also freeze avocado purée. Just add a tablespoon of

Fool-proof tips to eat more produce

Try these ideas and you may be surprised at how easily you add more fruits and vegetables to your diet.

▶ Put spinach on your sandwich instead of lettuce. A study found that people couldn't tell the difference, and spinach is more nutritious.

▶ Restaurants often pretty up your plate with parsley or kale. That's an arsenal of nutritional firepower that could be defending your health. Eat these garnishes right along with your meal.

▶ Add blueberries to pancake mix or muffin mix.

▶ Instead of butter or sour cream, top that baked potato with salsa.

▶ Substitute unsweetened applesauce for up to half the butter or oil called for in your baking recipes.

lemon juice, to prevent discoloration, for every two puréed avocados. Place the prepared purée in a freezer container with no more than a half-inch of airspace. Use the purée within four to five months.

The guide to going organic

Organically grown food is more popular then ever — but is it better for you? Studies show no significant differences in flavor, appearance, nutrient content, and bacterial contamination between organic and conventional food. However, organic food contains fewer pesticide residues, and organic meat may be somewhat safer. On the other hand, organic dairy products may not be worth the extra cost.

But there is more than safety and taste at stake. Keep in mind that organic farming is usually more environmentally sound and takes into account social issues — like fair trade and better treatment of labor — as well.

One of the biggest considerations in buying organic is the cost, which tends to be higher than that of conventional products. However, that trend may change as many mainstream grocery stores now offer their own brands of organic food.

It really comes down to personal choice. If you choose to shop for organic foods, federal labeling guidelines make sure you know what you're getting.

▶ 100 percent organic — no synthetic pesticides, herbicides, chemical fertilizers, antibiotics, hormones, additives, or preservatives.

▶ Organic — contains 95 percent or more organically produced ingredients.

▶ Made with organic ingredients — at least 70 percent of the product is organic.

If less than 70 percent of the product is organic, the word "organic" can't appear on the front of the package, but it can appear in the list of ingredients.

These national standards for organic foods give farmers clear production, handling, and processing guidelines and you, as a consumer, exact information about what you're buying.

For example, organic farmers can no longer use genetic engineering, radiation, sewage sludge for fertilizer, or any synthetic pesticide or fertilizer. In addition, animals used for meat, milk, eggs, etc., cannot receive hormones or antibiotics.

Look for the USDA organic label on a product to feel confident you're getting the most natural product possible.

Dodge pesticide dangers

When you bite into an apple, you know you're getting good nutrients like fiber, magnesium, potassium, and antioxidants. The one thing you may not count on is pesticides. But you can't be sure your produce is 100 percent pesticide-free. Even organically grown produce can contain some pesticide residues. According to the Environmental Working Group, the following fruits and vegetables tend to be the most and least contaminated.

Most contaminated	Least contaminated
peaches, strawberries, apples, spinach, nectarines, celery, pears, cherries, potatoes, sweet bell peppers, raspberries, and imported grapes	sweet corn, avocado, pineapples, cauliflower, mangoes, sweet peas, asparagus, onions, broccoli, bananas, kiwifruit, and papaya

That doesn't mean you should completely avoid certain fruits or vegetables. The health benefits of fruits and vegetables far outweigh any potential dangers of pesticides. So far, there has not been a definitive study showing how pesticide residues affect your health. Take these steps to lower your exposure.

Clean and cut away chemicals. Always scrub fruits and vegetables thoroughly before eating them. If you have any doubt about the skin's safety, remove it. Take advantage of canned fruits and vegetables as well. They tend to have fewer chemicals, probably because they are peeled before processing.

Broaden your selections. Eat fewer tainted foods by rotating them with others not on the list. Alternate eating spinach, kale, collards, and turnip greens, for instance. Munch on a rice cake instead of popcorn, and eat a variety of nuts. No food is guaranteed to be chemical-free, but you have a better chance of staying healthy if you eat a wide variety of foods.

Beat diabetes with bulgur

Bulgur, bulghur, or burghul — however you spell it, it's all the same, and it's all good. This deliciously healthy grain is made from whole-wheat berries or kernels that have been steamed, dried, and cracked. Some people confuse bulgur with cracked wheat, but bulgur is different since it's been pre-cooked.

This form of wheat is popular in Middle Eastern countries as the main ingredient in tabbouleh, a traditional salad of bulgur, parsley, cucumbers, tomatoes, olive oil, and lemon juice. It's also one of the oldest recorded types of foods — the Chinese may have eaten it as early as 2800 B.C. Lucky for us, bulgur is still around, because it has a hearty, nutty flavor, and is easy to cook. Don't forget how nutritious it is, either. Bulgur is a good source of insoluble fiber, protein, magnesium, iron, manganese, and B vitamins.

Add bulgur to your menu as a nice change from potatoes, and you'll cut your risk of diabetes, stroke, heart disease, and cancer. Look for boxes or bags of bulgur in your grocery or health food store.

Ditch diabetes. Large studies have consistently shown people eating at least three servings of whole grains a day have a 20 to 30 percent lower risk of type 2 diabetes than people who eat only three servings a week. Now evidence suggests high-fiber whole grains like bulgur may also help prevent metabolic syndrome, a risk factor for both type 2 diabetes and heart disease.

Fiber probably contributes to these protective benefits, but experts say there is more to it than that. Fiber from refined grains doesn't offer as much benefit as that from whole grain foods. Scientists suspect whole grains slow down the digestion of other foods and limit how much sugar your body absorbs from carbohydrates. Whole, unrefined grains also pack more nutrients, particularly magnesium, a mineral that helps control blood sugar.

The American Diabetes Association recommends getting at least 35 grams of fiber each day, but a recent study found eating 50 grams of fiber daily helped people with diabetes keep their blood sugar, insulin, and cholesterol all under control. A cup of cooked bulgur gets you well on your way toward reaching these goals with 8.2 grams of fiber. Besides that, it boasts loads of chromium, a mineral that makes insulin more effective. And since whole grain products tend to have a low glycemic index, bulgur is a good food to include in your diet.

Stop stroke. Try some tabbouleh or a side of bulgur pilaf instead of potatoes, and you'll add more than just variety to your diet. Recent research says eating whole grains like bulgur can reduce your risk of stroke.

Researchers at Brigham and Women's Hospital in Boston analyzed information on more than 75,000 women participating in the Nurses' Health Study. They found those who ate the highest amount of whole grains cut their risk of an ischemic stroke – the

Top sources of fiber	
Food	**Grams of fiber per cup**
Barley, pearled, raw	31.2
Bulgur, dry	25.6
Navy beans, boiled	19.1
Red kidney beans, canned	16.4
Split peas, boiled	16.3
Lentils, boiled	15.6
Pinto beans, boiled	15.4
Black beans, boiled	15.0
Wheat flour, whole-grain	14.6
Oat bran, raw	14.5
Dates, deglet noor	14.2
Refried beans, canned	13.4
Lima beans, large, boiled	13.2

kind caused by a blood clot to your brain – almost in half. Replacing refined grains like white rice and bread, cakes, biscuits, or pizza made from white flour, with whole grains like oatmeal, brown rice, bran, dark bread, and bulgur can mean a longer, healthier life.

Get a handle on heart disease. In most Middle Eastern or Asian countries, people get plenty of whole grains. But if you live in a western country, you are probably getting much less than nutrition experts recommend. Because of this, heart disease is widespread.

Whole grains like bulgur are good for your heart because they help control your weight, lower your blood pressure, and reduce bad LDL cholesterol levels while keeping your good HDL cholesterol steady. All this happens through a healthy combination of fiber, carbohydrates, essential fatty acids, and vitamins.

Study after study reports the more whole grains you eat, the lower your risk of developing heart disease. Louis Sullivan, M.D., former Secretary of the U.S. Department of Health and Human Services, takes the research seriously. "Increasing whole grain consumption could have a profound impact on the health of the nation," he says. "We could reduce the incidences of heart disease and cancer substantially."

Look for FDA-approved labels on certain products that say: "Diets rich in whole grain foods and other plant foods and low in total fat, saturated fat, and cholesterol may reduce the risk of heart disease and certain cancers."

Curtail cancer. The scientific community may not agree on how whole grains discourage cancer, but no one is arguing with the proof. If you were to look at all the research done on whole grains and cancer, you'd find positive results in 95 percent of the studies.

It may be the amount of fiber, antioxidants, or phytoestrogens in whole grains that do the trick. Or perhaps it's the way unprocessed grains help regulate your body's glucose levels. In any event, bulgur battles digestive system cancers, like colon cancer, and hormone-related cancers, such as breast and prostate cancer.

Remember, though, refining foods destroys many of the healthy components. Choose whole, unprocessed grain whenever possible.

Hit the road with fewer hassles

Living with diabetes can be hard enough, but traveling can really complicate things. Don't stay home for fear of being without your medicine or not finding the right food when you need it. People with diabetes can travel for fun or commute to a job — as long as they plan ahead. Even eating fast food can be healthy if you make the right choices. Michael F. Jacobson, Executive Director of Center for Science in the Public Interest and co-author of *Restaurant Confidential,* offers these tips for eating on the go.

Keep snacks in your car. Dangers of hypoglycemia, or low blood sugar, increase if you have to drive. Low blood sugar can make you feel weak and fatigued, as well as impair your thinking and eyesight. Know your own warning signs, and don't assume you'll be able to find a snack when you travel. Carry glucose tablets and extra rations, like Glucerna Meal Bars or DiabetX Snack Bars, with you.

Sneak a peek. Eating in a restaurant can be tricky, but many offer low-fat or other healthy meal options. Before you enter the

Fruit: an un-canny insight

You know fresh fruits can save your eyesight, fight cancer, and more, but sometimes you have to buy canned. No problem. To get the same benefits from canned fruit, make sure you buy the kind packed in its own juice, not in calorie-laden syrup.

Truth is, frozen and canned fruits generally have the same nutritional value as their fresh relatives. In some cases, they may even be healthier. Canned peaches, for instance, have only one-thousandth of the pesticides found on fresh peaches, possibly because they're peeled before processing.

restaurant, check the menu for healthy choices. Some chain restaurants carry nutritional information on their Web sites, so you can see your options before you arrive. If you can't find anything healthy, go to another place.

Avoid all-you-can eat buffets. It's not a deal if you save money, but load up on extra calories. If you do find yourself in an all-you-can-eat setting, limit yourself to two trips. Fill a dinner plate with fruits, salads, and other low-calorie vegetable dishes. Use a small salad plate for your second visit.

Watch portion sizes. There's no shame in leaving some food — and calories — on your plate. Ask for a doggie bag when you order, and put half your entrée in it before you start eating. That way, you won't overeat, and you'll have lunch for tomorrow. You can also split an entrée with a friend.

Consider going out for lunch instead of dinner. Lunch portions tend to be smaller — and cheaper. Or order a few appetizers, rather than a full meal.

Veg out. Look for dishes with fruits and vegetables. This might be harder than it sounds. "Chinese restaurants are one of the best places to get vegetables," Jacobson says. They usually cook to order, so you can ask them to use very little oil. And they don't use hydrogenated oil.

Skip fried foods. Just stay away from these diet disasters. "They are usually fried in hydrogenated shortening that is terrible for one's arteries," Jacobson says. Not to mention one's waistline.

Make requests. Don't be afraid to special order your meal. You're paying for it, after all. "When you're figuring out what to order, you should assume that you can ask for anything and let the waiter say you can't do it," says Jacobson. "So ask for the salad dressing on the side. Ask if you can substitute a side order of vegetables for a side order of French fries. Ask if they can bake it instead of frying it. The servers will generally try to do what you want."

Shop the supermarket. If you're out of snacks when low blood sugar strikes, stop by a grocery store for whole-grain bread and peanut butter or cheese. The local supermarket is also a great resource for quick, cheap meals if your travel accommodations include a kitchen. No kitchen? No problem. Grab some yogurt or a muffin for breakfast, order a sandwich from the deli counter for lunch, or even get a ready-made hot meal for dinner. Stocking up at the supermarket can also help you make healthy choices during the day.

Be careful with alcohol

Many studies suggest light to moderate drinking may protect you from heart disease and type 2 diabetes. While alcohol in general seems to dampen artery-harming inflammation, red wine takes the cake for protection. Experts say it may reduce your risk of type 2

Red meat raises red flags

Loading your dinner plate with red meat boosts levels of unhealthy fats in your blood and sets you up for type 2 diabetes. That's the latest from a new Harvard study. Red meat is chock full of a type of iron called heme. In this 20-year study of more than 85,000 women, diabetes risk rose with the amount of heme iron the women ate. Those who ate the most were 28 percent more likely to develop type 2 diabetes than those who ate the least heme.

Replacing that steak with a chicken breast, however, could help. A separate, small study found eating chicken in place of red meat improved kidney function in people with type 2 diabetes.

diabetes as well as improve insulin sensitivity and lower blood sugar levels in people who already have the disease.

That said, if you have neuropathy, a pancreas disease, or high levels of triglycerides, you should avoid alcohol. If you already suffer from neuropathy, it can make your symptoms worse, and even moderate drinking may raise your triglycerides if they are already high.

If you don't have these problems and your blood sugar is under good control, you can choose to have a drink now and then. Drink only in moderation – up to one drink a day for women or two for men. Large amounts can wreak havoc on your blood pressure. Remember to count the calories and carbohydrates. Avoid sweet liqueurs, and have your drink with food, not on an empty stomach.

Discover the joys of soy

Creamy tofu, soy milk and flour, tempeh and miso – their names may be unfamiliar to you, but these soy products are treasure troves of fiber, plant compounds, and a special soy protein that may help prevent both kidney and heart disease in people with type 2 diabetes.

Soybeans contain more protein than any other legume, and they are the only vegetable food whose protein is complete. That means there's no need to pair them with rice or pasta to get nutritional benefits. Soy protein may be big news for people with diabetes. Fourteen men with kidney disease and type 2 diabetes added a soy protein supplement to their diet for two months. The supplement boosted kidney function, raised "good" HDL cholesterol, and improved the ratio of HDL to "bad" LDL cholesterol.

Like other fruits and vegetables, soybeans have no cholesterol to clog your arteries. What they do have is lecithin, a plant compound that lowers cholesterol, helps the body digest fats, and prevents the buildup of fat in the arteries, as well as linolenic acid, one of the omega-3 fatty acids that helps reduce the risk of heart disease and stroke. New research in rats suggests a diet rich in black soy beans could lower triglycerides and both LDL and total cholesterol levels, plus help you lose weight. Soy beans are rich in fiber, too, both the soluble kind that cuts cholesterol and controls blood sugar and the insoluble kind that relieves constipation and helps fight stomach and colon cancers.

Yogurt made from soy milk also won big in a new lab study. Soy yogurt helped block enzymes involved in digesting carbohydrates, which helps slow down the absorption of glucose into your bloodstream. It also blocked the ACE-1 enzyme that narrows blood vessels, which could help lower your blood pressure. Soy yogurt flavored with

Flip a buckwheat flapjack

This grain may help lower blood sugar levels after meals, thanks to a compound known as D-chiro-inositol (D-CI). Canadian researchers gave buckwheat extract or a placebo to rats with type 1 diabetes after eating. Within two hours, the buckwheat rats had almost 20 percent lower blood sugar than those on placebo. In a separate study, eating biscuits made from buckwheat flower lowered blood sugar in people with diabetes.

Make a pasta salad or stir-fry with soba noodles, a Japanese pasta made from buckwheat. Or make a stack of flapjacks using buckwheat flour instead of white. It won't cure diabetes, but it could offer a cheap, simple, safe way to control blood sugar and cut the risk of heart, kidney, and nerve damage from diabetes.

blueberries was particularly powerful, with strawberry and peach soy yogurt close behind.

Nutritionists claim soy is the best vegetable food for maintaining normal blood sugar levels. You can try it yourself in moderation by snacking on soy yogurt, sipping soy milk, or serving up a side of black soy beans. You can even substitute one cup of soy flour plus one-fourth cup potato starch in place of one cup wheat flour in recipes. Just remember to account for the carbohydrates in these foods as part of your overall diabetes eating plan.

Making good use of multivitamins

Foods are by far the healthiest, most natural way to get quality nutrition. Having diabetes does not change your nutritional needs, but aging does. As your body ages, it may need more of certain nutrients than you can get from food, particularly calcium and vitamins D and B12. Certain medications may also cause deficiencies. For instance, research links the diabetes drug metformin with low blood levels of vitamin B12.

Angle for more apricots

This one sweet little fruit is loaded with as many nutrients as you'll find in your multivitamin — beta carotene, iron, fiber, vitamin C, several B vitamins, lycopene, potassium, magnesium, and copper. That makes apricots the nutrient super-hero of the produce aisle. Eat them often to battle cancer, high blood pressure, memory loss, and cataracts. You'll get even more nutrient power concentrated in dried apricots and can enjoy them out of season in jams, spreads, and nectars.

Your best bet is to fill your nutritional bill with food, then discuss dietary supplements with your doctor. Too much of certain vitamins or minerals can be toxic or mask other illnesses. If you decide to take a multivitamin, choose one without iron. Men and post-menopausal women don't usually need the extra iron, and too much of this mineral can cause constipation and may increase your risk of colorectal cancer.

Pucker up to smooth out spikes

Honey may help you catch more flies, but vinegar chases off disease. This acidic juice seems to slow down the digestion of food, evening out blood sugar spikes after a meal. In a recent study, people who were insulin-resistant – a condition that can lead to diabetes – drank a mixture of apple cider vinegar and water before eating. They saw their after-meal blood sugar drop 34 percent compared to those who drank a placebo, and they experienced smaller spikes in insulin and glucose.

Evidence suggests just three teaspoons of vinegar can lower your after-meal blood sugar as much as 30 percent, while adding only two calories – and lots of flavor – to any meal. You can lower your blood sugar level by adding tangy lemon juice to your foods, too, since it's also acidic. So drop a slice of lemon in your water or splash a dash of red wine vinegar on your salads for better sugar control.

Cooking tricks tame heart villain

It's not what you cook that's important. It's how you cook it. Why? Chemicals called advanced glycation end products (AGEs). These components form naturally when foods containing sugars, fats, and proteins are cooked at high temperatures for a long time.

Although scientists have known about AGEs for a while, they only recently discovered the danger to people with diabetes. In fact, according to the latest research from New York's Mount Sinai School of Medicine, AGEs could be a major reason why diabetes sufferers face such a high risk for heart disease. The researchers suspect AGEs cause their immune systems to overreact, which could eventually damage blood vessels.

The good news – you can control the amount of AGEs you consume. Follow these tips to lower the number of AGEs in your food.

Limit animal foods. Out of more than 200 foods tested for AGEs, animal foods cooked at high temperatures topped the list, especially those high in fat and protein like meat, cheese, and egg yolks.

Change the way you cook. High-humidity cooking methods, like boiling and steaming, could produce fewer AGEs in your food. Quick cooking at low heat, like stir-frying, is another healthy option. Just remember – baking, grilling, and broiling could be harmful to your blood vessels.

Though the Mount Sinai research is in its early stages, it can't hurt to follow these recommendations now. They could also protect you from kidney disease and other complications.

How to pick the freshest foods

You hear all sorts of advice about which foods you should eat, but what about the quality of the food you buy? Pay attention to any product's "sell by" date, then consider these suggestions before adding items to your shopping cart.

Meat and poultry. The color of meat indicates its freshness. Beef should be a bright red, while young veal and pork are grayish-pink, and older veal is a darker pink. When it comes to poultry, look for meaty birds with creamy white to yellow skin. Watch out for bruises, tiny feathers, and torn or dry skin.

5-a-day now minimum for benefit

Five servings per day used to be the accepted standard for fruits and vegetables. But now a group that includes the National Cancer Institute and the American Cancer Society says that should only be a minimum. Active women need seven servings a day; active men need nine.

You may be closer to these recommendations than you think. A serving is only about as much as will fit in the palm of your hand. That's a medium stalk of broccoli, a half-dozen baby carrots, or a small banana. Other single servings are:

▶ one-half cup of cooked vegetables, diced fruit or vegetables, or cooked beans

▶ one-fourth cup of dried fruit

▶ a full cup of raw salad greens

▶ 6 ounces of 100-percent fruit or vegetable juice

Fish. A fresh filet or steak will have firm flesh without any gaps in it. If it's fresh, a fish with its head will have bright eyes and red gills. Avoid any fish with patches of slimy or dried-out flesh, blood spots, or other unappealing marks. Fresh fish won't smell fishy either.

Produce. Examine fruits or vegetables for firmness and color. Avoid bruised or wilted produce, which may be past its peak. Fresh, locally grown produce may pack more nutritional bang for your buck. The faster it gets from the field to your plate, the more vitamins and minerals you get to enjoy.

Eat to overcome 'silent killer'

About one in four Americans have metabolic syndrome, or Syndrome X, a combination of symptoms that raises your risk of diabetes, heart disease, and stroke. (To learn about this condition, read *What is prediabetes?* in the *Blood Sugar Basics* chapter.)

Dr. Gerald Reaven is the Stanford University professor who first discovered and named metabolic syndrome. He recently published his findings from four decades of revolutionary research in the book *Syndrome X: The Silent Killer.*

At the heart of this work is an eating plan designed especially to battle metabolic syndrome. Follow it, and you may control your insulin, lower your low-density lipoprotein (LDL) cholesterol levels, and lose weight. Amazingly, you'll also find the plan easy, delicious, and nutritious.

Reverse the ratio of carbs. Reaven's eating plan stands traditional medical wisdom on its head. For years, health experts recommended a low-fat, high-carbohydrate diet for a healthy heart. They believed carbohydrates should make up to 60 percent of your daily calories. That way, they'll replace saturated fats and keep your LDL cholesterol in check. But according to Reaven, all those carbohydrates can be disastrous if you have metabolic syndrome.

"It's so obvious," Reaven says. "If you eat more carbohydrates, you need more insulin. And the more insulin resistant you are, the more insulin you need." When you eat carbohydrates, your body breaks them down into simple sugars. Insulin's job is to wrangle up this sugar as it enters your bloodstream and lead it to your cells. The cells then take it up and use it for energy, and your blood sugar decreases. "Insulin acts to put carbohydrates in the right places," Reaven says.

If you have metabolic syndrome, however, your cells don't take in the sugar. Your body releases more and more insulin until, finally, the cells absorb the glucose, and your blood sugar drops. But the stress of all that insulin can damage the linings of your arteries and put you one step closer to heart disease.

Reaven's plan leaves carbohydrates as only 45 percent of your daily calories. Don't fret about the kind of carbohydrates. "Not as long as you're eating real food," suggests Reaven. Whole grains, fruits, and vegetables are all fine, as long as you maintain the 45-percent ratio.

Eat more "good" fat. Reaven's solution to this crisis may sound off-the-wall — trade in those extra carbohydrates for fat. It's not so crazy an idea, since it's the monounsaturated fatty acids (MUFAs) and polyunsaturated fatty acids (PUFAs) he's talking about. These are the "good" fats that don't increase your LDL cholesterol. And unlike carbohydrates, they won't raise your blood sugar.

Make these good fats 30 to 35 percent of your daily diet. Meanwhile, keep the unhealthy saturated fat to no more than 5 to 10 percent. "That accomplishes the same advantage for LDL cholesterol," Reaven states, "but it does it without the untoward effect of making you make more insulin."

To meet your daily ration of good fats, include sources of both polyunsaturated fatty acids and monounsaturated fatty acids. Fish, flaxseed and flaxseed oil, canola oil, walnuts, and seeds are all loaded with PUFAs. For MUFAs, try olive and canola oils, peanuts, almonds, cashews, pecans, and avocados. As for saturated fats, steer clear of red meat, whole-fat dairy products, eggs, coconut oil, and processed and fried foods.

Steady your protein intake. Believe it or not, protein can increase your insulin just like carbohydrates. So Reaven's plan keeps protein at a minimum — 15 percent of your calories. That might disappoint you if you're a fan of high-protein diets. But considering the roller coaster ride protein-rich diets may send your blood sugar on, not to mention the saturated fat they usually contain, they may only make your insulin resistance, heart disease, and other symptoms of metabolic syndrome worse.

In the long-run, that could be fatal. Your pancreas, which is your body's insulin factory, could break down after years of pumping out too much of the hormone. That leaves you with type 2 diabetes. Or you could be looking at a heart attack after all that damage to your blood vessels.

No wonder people listen when Reaven talks. If you want to follow his advice, work with your doctor to incorporate Reaven's guidelines into your own eating habits.

Diabetes danger foods

If you think pizza is your friend, recent findings suggest you had better think again. One study of diabetic volunteers who ate pizza for dinner showed much higher blood sugar levels during that night's sleep, even though levels were controlled after the meal. Researchers aren't sure what ingredient in the pizza caused this blood sugar increase. Because of this danger, the delicious pie is probably a better choice for lunch than dinner.

Oysters-on-the-half-shell are another favorite treat, but they can be deadly. Shellfish like oysters, clams, and mussels feed by straining water through their systems, which makes them more likely to pick up dangerous bacteria in the ocean. These bacteria can cause food poisoning and even blood poisoning when shellfish are eaten raw. This is dangerous for anyone, but it poses a special threat for people with diabetes. Fortunately, you can kill these bacteria by cooking shellfish thoroughly.

Wondering about sushi? Raw fin fish can contain its own kind of parasites and bacteria. Freezing kills the parasites, but only thorough cooking kills all the bacteria. Because of the special risk, people with diabetes should never eat raw or undercooked seafood of any kind.

Should you go low-carb?

Carbohydrates have more effect on blood sugar than any other nutrient. So does it help to limit your carbs? A recent Temple University study of 10 obese people with type 2 diabetes found that a strict low-carb diet helped them lose weight and improve blood sugar levels. However, the study was small and strictly controlled, and the long-term effects of such a diet — high in protein and fat and low in fiber — remain unknown.

In fact, a recent Harvard study shows that the iron from red meat can lead to type 2 diabetes. And there are concerns about a high-protein diet's effect on your kidneys — not to mention your heart and arteries. Your best bet is to talk to your doctor before beginning a low-carbohydrate, high-protein diet.

Another problem if you have diabetes is getting too much protein. Meat and dairy products are full of this nutrient. While protein is a necessary building block for the growth and repair of your body, too much of a good thing can be dangerous. Any protein your body can't use has to be eliminated, and this means extra work for your already-hard-working kidneys.

Also, because many sources of protein are high in saturated fat and cholesterol, people who eat excess amounts of protein are at higher risk of heart disease. Ask your doctor how much protein you should eat every day, and follow his advice carefully.

Eat right to live longer

Don't think of diabetes in terms of what you can't eat. Think of what you can eat. Make these delicious, healthy food substitutions for a longer life.

Instead of	Eat
red meat, hot dogs, bacon, sausage	poultry, fish
white bread	bread made from "stone-ground" flour
refined white flour	buckwheat flour
highly processed foods	fresh whole legumes, fruits, and vegetables
sugary drinks like sodas	low-fat milk, water
meat	beans
cornflakes	raisin bran
orange juice	whole orange
white rice	brown rice

ACE this eating plan to control sugar

You no longer have to nibble on carrot sticks instead of a cookie just because you have diabetes. The American Association of Clinical Endocrinologists (AACE) now says up to 10 percent of your daily calories can come from sugar — if you adjust for the extra calories.

A task force from the AACE and the American College of Endocrinology revised the original 1994 guidelines for people with diabetes. Their aim is to help keep blood glucose as close to normal as possible and to avoid long-term complications of the disease.

Lower your target blood sugar. Experts now say if you have diabetes you should strive for blood sugar of less than 110 mg/dl before a meal and less than 140 after. If these numbers seem lower than you remember, it's because they are. Keeping tighter control over your blood sugar will pay off with fewer complications later in life. Stick with these new guidelines if you hope to avoid kidney disease, blindness, amputations, and heart disease.

Get your ratios right. The AACE recommends your diet include 10 to 20 percent protein, 55 to 60 percent carbohydrates, and less than 30 percent fat. Keep salt in your diet to less than 3 grams a day.

Control your calories. Just losing 10 to 20 pounds can make a big difference in your blood sugar, blood pressure, and blood fats. You don't even have to reach your ideal weight – simply start by keeping this much weight off. Although this information isn't new, the AACE thought it was important enough to repeat.

Be careful with alcohol. The guidelines still say you should be cautious about drinking. Avoid it altogether if you have neuropathy, a pancreas disease, or high triglyceride levels. If you don't have these problems and you keep your blood sugar under control, you can choose to have a drink now and then. Be sure to discuss it with your doctor first.

Delicious way to get tough on cholesterol

If your cholesterol numbers fall within the healthy range, but you have diabetes, you can't relax. The American Diabetes Association suggests you keep your LDL (bad) cholesterol under 100 milligrams per deciliter (mg/dl) and your HDL (good) cholesterol above 45 mg/dl for men and 55 mg/dl for women. These guidelines are tougher than those recommended for the general population. Yet research proves if you work hard to lower your LDL cholesterol, you'll reduce your risk of heart disease complications.

Tomatoes may be a secret weapon in this battle. When unstable molecules – called free radicals – attack LDL particles, the damaged particles become oxidized LDL. "When LDL is oxidized, it leads to the formation of plaque in the vessel – known as atherosclerosis," explains Dr. Joye Willcox, a registered dietician and owner of the private weight management practice Healthy Diets, Inc. As more plaques form, the walls of these arteries become thicker, constricting the flow of blood. Eventually, an artery may get clogged enough to cause a heart attack. But that doesn't have to happen.

Arm yourself with antioxidants

You've heard that antioxidants are good for you, but you may be surprised to learn just how severely you need them. When your body processes the oxygen you breathe, unstable compounds called free radicals are created at the same time. These villains stalk through your body hunting for electrons to steal from healthy cells in order to become stable. When they succeed, they leave the cell irreversibly damaged. Over time that damage adds up. Researchers have linked free radical damage to more than 200 diseases, including cataracts, diabetes, heart disease, and some cancers.

Antioxidants are mighty nutrients that combine with free radicals to render them stable – and harmless. Research proves you can raise your levels of antioxidants by eating more fruits and vegetables.

Willcox and other scientists think something special in tomatoes may help prevent plaque. The most likely candidates are antioxidant compounds like vitamin C and lycopene. "Antioxidants provide protection in the inner layer of blood vessels to prevent LDL cholesterol from being oxidized," says Willcox.

That may mean something as convenient as tomato juice could stop your cholesterol from oxidizing and sticking to your artery walls. You may be able to stop plaque and clogged arteries before they can even get started.

Slice your risk. Some studies suggest the tomato's most famous antioxidant – lycopene – could be the hero that rescues hearts.

▶ Dutch researchers examined the blood vessels and blood of 108 elderly people. The higher the amount of lycopene they found in a person's blood, the lower the risk of atherosclerosis seemed to be – especially for smokers or former smokers.

▶ A study of more than 1,000 men in Finland found those with low levels of lycopene in their blood had thicker artery walls – a sign of atherosclerosis.

▶ According to American research, older women with more lycopene in their blood may have up to 34 percent less risk of heart disease than those with the lowest lycopene levels.

▶ Australian researchers found drinking at least 8 ounces of clarified, or filtered, tomato juice a day lowered the risk for atherosclerosis, heart attack, and stroke in people with type 2 diabetes.

▶ In another clinical study, drinking about 17 ounces a day for a month kept cholesterol from oxidizing and attaching to artery walls – a process that hardens and blocks your arteries. This amount of tomato juice nearly tripled people's levels of lycopene, a carotenoid proven to guard against heart attacks.

Choose foods, not supplements. Willcox and her colleagues examined the research on what lycopene can do without help from other nutrients. They found some studies where lycopene reduced LDL oxidation and others where it did not. Even studies on other tomato antioxidants had the same mixed results. Yet, research on whole fruits and vegetables consistently showed more promise. Willcox and her colleagues concluded that eating tomatoes and tomato products could be good protection for your heart.

Cook 'em up right. "Cooking appears to increase the absorption of lycopene," says Willcox. That means you may get more lycopene from processed tomato products – especially those with a little oil. For example, the oil in tomato paste and tomato sauces helps your body take in more lycopene. For best results, stick with healthy oils like olive oil, and avoid saturated fats and trans fats. "One cup of tomato sauce or two cups of tomato juice would provide approximately 40 milligrams of lycopene," Willcox says. That amount of daily lycopene from food may be enough to affect the oxidation of LDL cholesterol, according to one study.

Tomatoes are not for everyone, though. If you have heartburn or acid reflux, tomatoes could make your discomfort worse. Some experts also suspect tomatoes may aggravate arthritis.

Head off heart attacks from hidden fat

Watch out for a little-known danger that may sneak up on you while you are busy focusing on your cholesterol. Triglycerides, an equally dangerous fat, may be just waiting to strike. One study found your risk of having a heart attack is three times greater if you have high triglycerides compared to those with normal levels.

Triglycerides are fats that provide most of the fuel for your body. You get some from the fat in your diet, and your liver makes the rest from the carbohydrates you eat. Like all fats, they are necessary, within limits, for good health. But studies have found a link between elevated triglyceride levels and heart disease. And high triglycerides and high LDL cholesterol together deal a double whammy to your heart's health.

Tempt your tastebuds

Healthy foods can taste just as exciting and yummy as fattening ones. Try these surprisingly clever tricks for more tempting and flavorful veggies.

▸ Top corn or black beans with salsa or a dash of hot sauce.

▸ Add garlic to mashed potatoes.

▸ Make a grated carrot salad.

▸ Add a dash of nutmeg to spinach dishes.

▸ Microwave a sweet potato with ground cloves or cinnamon on top.

▸ Add sliced or diced vegetables to meatloaf or scrambled eggs.

▸ Steam broccoli and sprinkle on Parmesan cheese.

On the other hand, the combination of low triglycerides and high HDL cholesterol is a plus. It puts you at less risk for heart disease even if your LDL cholesterol is high. Unfortunately, a good HDL level alone won't protect you if your triglycerides are out of sight. And if triglyceride problems run in your family, you're more likely to die from a heart attack even when your blood cholesterol is normal, says Melissa A. Austin, Ph.D., a researcher at the University of Washington. She and her colleagues looked at the medical histories of more than 100 families over 20 years and found that high triglyceride levels could predict heart attacks years in advance.

Fortunately, a few simple changes may be all you need to get your triglycerides under control. One of the most important things you can do for your heart is to keep your weight in a healthy range by balancing the calories you take in with those you burn. Your body converts extra calories to triglycerides and stores them, increasing your chances of heart disease. The chapter *Slimming Down: Simple steps to reverse diabetes* will guide you in reaching your goals. Next, stop smoking and start getting regular exercise. You'll find fun activities in the chapter *Active Living: Shape up to shake high blood sugar.* Last, but not least, rethink the way you eat, without sacrificing taste or starving yourself.

Limit sugar and white breads. Eat more whole grains, and keep sweets to a minimum in your diet. Refined carbohydrates – like baked goods made with white flour – and simple carbohydrates – like sugar, honey, corn syrup, and molasses – can raise your triglycerides.

Eat less saturated fat. Avoid fatty cuts of meats and full-fat dairy products. But don't cut your total fat to less than 15 percent of your daily calories. According to the American Heart Association, going lower can increase your triglycerides and reduce your HDL cholesterol, just the opposite of what you want.

The latest government guidelines on cholesterol recommend keeping your fat intake under 35 percent of your daily calories. Replace saturated fats with healthier ones – like the monounsaturated fats found in olive, canola, and peanut oils, as well as avocados and nuts.

Focus on fiber. Eating whole grains, dried beans and other fibrous vegetables, and fruits with their skins will help lower triglycerides. But don't count on the same good results from fiber supplements.

Eat more fatty fish. Salmon, albacore, blue fin tuna, sardines, lake trout, and mackerel are all healthy sources of omega-3 fatty acids. These, and fish oil supplements as well, can help lower triglycerides.

Watch your alcohol intake. Although moderate drinking seems to benefit your heart in some ways, it can also increase your triglycerides if they are already high. If you drink, stay at or below the recommended daily limit of two drinks – containing one-half ounce of pure alcohol – if you are a male and one drink if you are a female.

If you find these lifestyle changes don't lower your triglycerides to 150 or below – considered normal under the new government guidelines – talk to your doctor about medications that can help. Besides putting you at risk for heart disease, high triglycerides could be a sign of diabetes, an under-active thyroid, kidney disease, or some other serious health problem.

Reverse diabetes with no-hunger diet

Reverse your diabetes simply by giving up animal protein. That's the message from a recent study.

Researchers tried a new diet plan on 51 people with diabetes who could no longer control their disease with high doses of medicine or insulin. The diet allowed no sugar and only one serving of animal protein – such as meat or fish – every other day. The participants ate vegetable protein to make up for the missing calories and continued on their usual medicines. Those who stuck to the diet reportedly liked it because they didn't skip meals or cut calories so they weren't hungry.

After six months, the people who followed the diet had amazing results. Although they didn't lose weight, their blood fats and sugar levels returned to normal or near normal. Some were able to stop taking medicine, and others only needed half as much. The researchers conclude that a diet low in animal protein and sugar can reverse diabetes or improve metabolism so medicines can work.

If you'd like to try the diet, get permission from your doctor first. You'll have to avoid sugar and substitute vegetable protein like tofu, nuts, or legumes for meat at least three nights a week. And remember, eggs count as animal protein. Eat meatless soups, sandwiches, or salads for lunch, and include whole-grain cereals in your breakfast menu.

KO heart disease in 6 easy steps

As a person with diabetes, defending yourself against heart disease is a matter of life or death. Diabetes quietly but steadily damages your heart and blood vessels – and increases your odds of having a fatal heart attack or stroke. In fact, women with diabetes are almost three times more likely to die within a few years of a heart attack than are non-diabetic women.

Heart disease is the leading cause of death in the United States and other developed countries, but it's rapidly becoming a world-wide problem. But you don't have to take these statistics lying down. It's one disease you can do something about, no matter where you live.

Because heart disease is such a serious problem, the American Heart Association (AHA) issues dietary guidelines to help people battle it. The AHA recommendations include eating at least five servings of various fruits and vegetables daily; six or more servings of grains daily; two or more servings of fish weekly; and limiting your intake of saturated fat, cholesterol, salt, and alcohol.

Fill up on fiber. Do you want an easy way to follow the American Heart Association's recommendations for a heart-healthy diet? Just add two bowls of high-fiber cereal to your diet every day.

In a recent study, men who ate two servings of high-fiber cereal each day – one for breakfast and one later in the day as a snack – changed their diets enough to meet the AHA's recommendations for fat and cholesterol. Eating cereal for breakfast meant they ate fewer fatty breakfast foods, like omelets, pastries, and breakfast sandwiches. And some of the men ate cereal as an after-dinner snack, instead of their usual bowl of ice cream.

Researchers didn't tell them to make any changes except adding the cereal to their regular diets, but the men found that they automatically ate fewer fatty foods because the fiber was so filling.

Because fiber helps lower cholesterol, the AHA recommends eating soluble fiber, found in foods such as oatmeal, oat bran, rice bran, beans, barley, citrus fruits, strawberries, and apples, as well as insoluble fiber found in whole wheat breads and cereals, brown rice and many fruits and vegetables.

Fight back with folate. Homocysteine, an amino acid your body produces as a by-product of protein metabolism, could be as damaging to your heart and blood vessels as cholesterol. Scientists have found that people with heart disease, strokes, or clogged arteries in their legs are much more likely to have high levels of homocysteine in their blood.

Luckily, it's easy to fight homocysteine with the right foods. Folate and other B vitamins break down homocysteine in your body. That's why people with high levels of folate usually have low levels of homocysteine.

To boost your folate level, eat lots of green leafy vegetables, beans, citrus fruits, and fortified cereals and breads.

Fish for more omega-3. If you want to keep your heart healthy, eat fish more often. A large study on male doctors found those who ate at least one fish meal a week were 52 percent less likely to die from a sudden heart attack than those who ate fish less than once a month.

Omega-3 fatty acids are the heart heroes in fish. Research indicates that omega-3 can lower your blood pressure, reduce the stickiness of your blood, and help regulate your heartbeat. Fatty fish, such as tuna and salmon, contain lots of omega-3. If you're not a big fan of fish, you can also get omega-3 in flaxseed oil and some green leafy vegetables, like spinach and kale.

Bake with barley flour

Barley flour has more than three times the fiber of wheat flour, but it doesn't have the kind of gluten to make baked goods rise properly. For best results, mix it with regular wheat flour. For yeast breads, substitute barley flour for about a quarter of your total flour. For cookies and quick breads, use half and half.

Up the ante with antioxidants. The AHA recommends you eat at least five servings of fruits and vegetables every day. Fresh fruits and vegetables are loaded with natural compounds called antioxidants that may prevent LDL cholesterol from becoming oxidized.

Dr. Lori J. Mosca, director of preventive cardiology research and education at the University of Michigan, says, "When a fat such as LDL undergoes oxidation, it is more prone to collect in blood vessels to form plaque. Over time, the plaque narrows the blood vessels, or unleashes a blood clot, which can result in a heart attack or stroke. When LDL is not oxidized, it does not seem to cause problems." These powerful antioxidants, in particular, can help keep your heart healthy.

- ▶ Vitamin C. Besides protecting cells from oxidation, vitamin C also helps keep blood vessels open wide. Citrus fruits, strawberries, cantaloupe, tomatoes, brussels sprouts, and broccoli provide beneficial amounts of vitamin C.

- ▶ Flavonoids. If you shoot for the AHA's recommendation of five or more servings of fruits and vegetables every day, you'll easily get a healthy dose of heart friendly flavonoids. These compounds protect your heart by preventing the build-up of plaque in your arteries. One study found that broccoli was particularly protective. Tea, onions, and apples came out the heart-protective winners in another study.

Switch to unsaturated fat. If you often shout, "Cheeseburger, fries, and a chocolate shake, please," into a speaker from your car, you're a perfect example of why heart disease is the leading cause of death in most developed countries. People eat too much fat.

Yet, not all fats are created equal when it comes to keeping your heart healthy. Fats born on sunny Mediterranean shores may actually do your heart good. People who eat a typical Mediterranean diet rich in olive oil are less likely to have heart disease.

To protect your heart from harmful fats, eat less saturated fat, found in meat, dairy products, and some vegetable oils, like coconut oil and palm oil.

Veg out. Studies find that vegetarians are less likely to develop heart disease than meat eaters. Dr. Dean Ornish's well-known program for reversing heart disease includes following a very low-fat vegetarian diet. The program also includes getting regular exercise, managing stress, and stopping smoking.

If you decide to follow Dr. Ornish's program, try it at least three or four weeks. It takes that long to break bad habits and establish a new, healthy lifestyle. For details on following this special diet plan, see *Popular diets: what works, what doesn't* in the chapter *Slimming Down: Simple steps to reverse diabetes.*

Beat two diseases with one humble grain

What do Spartacus and Budweiser have in common? Barley – the hearty grain that gladiators ate to give them strength and that breweries use to make beer.

Barley's popularity and status as a health food goes back thousands of years. Greeks cultivated it as long ago as 7000 B.C., and ancient Chinese, Egyptians, and Romans made it an important part of their diets. People also used barley to treat boils, stomach disorders, and urinary tract infections.

Today, barley crops up mostly in soups, cereal, beer, and animal feed. But its ability to fight heart disease and diabetes should earn it a more prominent place in your diet. After all, barley practically overflows with fiber and contains key minerals like potassium, phosphorus, magnesium, and iron.

Loading up on soups and cereal made with barley isn't the only way to get more of this great grain. Next time you're baking, try sifting some barley flour into the mixing bowl. Or add some barley to your rice to create a more fiber-rich meal.

Think of it as entering the arena to battle the enemies of good health.

Conquers cholesterol. Behind every healthy food, there is a healthy ingredient. In the case of barley, the behind-the-scenes dynamo is a form of soluble fiber called beta glucan. Powered by beta glucan, barley has shown time and again it can lower cholesterol. And remember, when you cut artery-clogging cholesterol, you also cut your risk of heart disease. Even in forms as different as barley flour, oil, muesli, or pasta, the results are the same.

As food travels through your body, low-density lipoprotein (LDL) particles carry cholesterol to cells, where it can do damage. High-density lipoprotein (HDL) particles pick up the cholesterol and whisk it to your liver, which converts it to bile and gets rid of it. This process is called "reverse cholesterol transport."

Dr. Barbara Schneeman, a researcher with the USDA's Agricultural Research Service and professor of agricultural and environmental sciences at the University of California-Davis, believes barley affects cholesterol levels through its viscosity, or stickiness.

Because beta glucan is sticky, it slows down the movement of food through your stomach and small intestine. That gives the

HDL particles more time to pick up cholesterol, reducing the chances it will be absorbed later. "It's slowing lipid absorption and giving more time for reverse cholesterol transport to happen," Schneeman explains.

Balances out blood pressure. Not only does barley have more fiber than any other grain, it also contains potassium and magnesium – two of the top minerals for fighting high blood pressure. This combination may also lower your chance of stroke. In fact, the Food and Drug Administration (FDA) recently decided to allow foods meeting specific requirements for potassium, sodium, fat, and cholesterol to advertise they reduce the risk of high blood pressure and stroke. You may see a claim like this on your next package of barley.

Defeats diabetes. Because of barley's effect on cholesterol and other heart concerns, you might have guessed it would be a good food for people with diabetes. Experts specifically recommend a high-fiber diet with both soluble and cereal fiber. Barley fits the bill.

Schneeman again points to viscosity as a possible factor. Instead of glucose rushing through the blood, demanding insulin all at once, it oozes through at a snail's pace. This affects the demand for insulin by "slowing it down; spreading it out a bit," she says.

Manages weight. Obesity seriously raises your risk for a variety of health problems, including heart disease. But the fiber in barley can help you lose weight. Here's how.

A certain hormone in your gut, cholecystokinin (CCK), is associated with feelings of fullness. When people eat a low-fat diet, their CCK levels go up, then back down to normal, or fasting, level. When they eat barley, their CCK still goes up after the meal, but it never makes it all the way back down to fasting level. That means you'll probably feel more full after a barley meal. And if you feel full, you're less likely to overeat and put on unwanted pounds.

"Fiber intake doesn't cause weight loss. Energy restriction causes weight loss," Schneeman stresses. "The challenge for most people is to stay in control between meals. If something like fiber promotes a little bit of a feeling of fullness, it can help in that phase."

You can eat barley plain or serve it in soups and casseroles. Pearl barley – the most common barley product – has been polished to remove the hard outer shell. Serve it as a side dish in place of rice or pasta.

Slimming Down

Simple steps to reverse diabetes

Focus on a healthier body

You look good and feel energetic when you maintain a trim figure, but your health is an even more important reason to watch your weight. Doctors used to think people older than 55 didn't gain and, in fact, gradually lost pounds. But that doesn't always hold true. Obesity, or excess body fat, is growing faster among seniors than any other group.

Experts say extra weight hurts your health even more than smoking or heavy drinking. It increases your risk for diabetes, heart disease, osteoarthritis, stroke, high blood pressure, sleep apnea and other breathing problems, gallbladder disease, and some forms of cancer.

Type 2 diabetes in particular is related to carrying excess weight. As developing countries become more prosperous, rates of diabetes among their citizens tend to grow along with waistlines. But experts say half the world's cases of type 2 diabetes could be prevented by taking the one step of losing a small amount of weight.

If you're overweight, diabetic, and have visited your doctor lately, she may have suggested you try to shed some pounds. It's easy for a doctor to say, "Lose weight and control your blood sugar." What then? Many doctors don't give their patients good advice on how to lose weight and aren't up to date on the latest nutritional standards. A Washington state study found two-thirds of the doctors surveyed wanted more information to help patients manage their weight. Perhaps because they are unsure of what to say, many doctors don't bring up the subject of weight – even to people who are obese.

The good news is that small steps on the road to a slimmer you can make a big difference. If you are overweight, starting on a healthy weight-loss plan now may add years to your life. Take heart from these happy facts.

▶ Researchers found that just trying to lose weight – even if you don't succeed – can help you live longer. The key may be that, in trying to lose weight, you are likely to eat foods that are more nutritious and practice a healthier lifestyle.

▶ Taking a 30-minute daily walk and losing 10 or 15 pounds can help you avoid type 2 diabetes and add years to your life – even if you lose just one pound a year. That's equal to cutting just 10 calories a day. The key is keeping the weight off over time.

▶ You may be able to lose weight without even trying. At the University of Kentucky College of Medicine, 24 men ate canned beans – a good source of fiber – for three weeks. Even while consuming the same total calories, the men lost weight. This 50-cent meal lowered their cholesterol, too.

You can win the battle and lose the bulge. Read on for more great ideas on keeping your weight in check.

Slow and steady wins the weight-loss race

If you're thinking of jumping into a fast weight-loss diet, slow down. A "quick fix" won't work in the long run. Overeating is likely to follow, taking you right back to where you started. In fact, if you want to lose weight, starting a strict diet is probably the last thing you should do.

Your best plan of action is to make moderate changes in your diet with the goal of losing one or two pounds a week. Decide how many calories you are presently eating, on average, each day. Then take steps to reduce that amount by 500 to 1,000 calories.

As a rule, experts don't recommend eating less than 1,200 calories. "However," says registered dietitian Kimberly Gaddy, "folks that need quick weight loss for health or motivation reasons – typically folks who need to lose 60 or more pounds – may need to be on a calorie level of less than 1,200 for faster initial weight reduction."

Going lower than 800 calories can be dangerous – especially for people over 50. Have your doctor evaluate your risks and benefits

Beware of villain lurking in produce aisle

Don't be tempted by that carton of caramel dipping sauce sitting next to the apples in the produce aisle. It may seem like the perfect accompaniment, but just two tablespoons of that sweet treat has 110 calories and 14 grams of sugar. And that's the light version. Stick with the natural sweetness of the apple instead.

of a very low calorie diet before you take this gamble. No matter what your age, you need medical supervision if you are on a diet this severe.

"It is important to focus on long-term behavior change," says Gaddy. If you want to keep your new size and shape, you have to form new habits. The key is to exercise and eat a healthy diet, taking in no more calories than you burn. One thing's for sure – a positive attitude and a solid plan can help. Check out these weight-loss strategies that work for a lifetime.

Strive for five. How do you go about cutting fat from your diet? Penn State researchers recently examined the strategies of 65 successful dieters. All were at least 50 years old and had stuck to their fat-busting diets for at least five years. Here are their top five secrets to success.

▶ Savor summer fruit. Eat more cantaloupes, watermelon, peaches, plums, and nectarines.

▶ Eat more vegetables and grains. Make room for sweet potatoes, squash, beans, cooked greens, mixed salads, broccoli, rice, and noodles.

▶ Cut back on recreational foods. Say goodbye to cookies, chocolate candy, chips, crackers, doughnuts, and ice cream, and say hello to low-fat pizza and desserts.

▶ Decrease cooking fat. Eat less cream or meat sauces, butter, margarine, oil, cream soups, ground meat, cheese, pizza, fried chicken, french fries, and mayonnaise-based salads. Pop popcorn without oil, and eat tuna without mayonnaise.

▶ Use fat-modified foods. Stock up on low-fat salad dressing, mayonnaise, and spreads. Remove the skin from chicken, and trim the fat from beef. Drink low-fat milk.

These simple strategies allowed the dieters in the Penn State study to slash their fat intake nearly in half. But it didn't happen overnight. In most cases, these lifelong weight watchers made changes to their diets gradually.

Set goals. Think of losing weight as a journey between where you are now and where you want to be. Wandering aimlessly and hoping to reach your destination probably won't work. You need a map.

Track your progress by setting short-term goals and monitoring yourself. When you reach one goal, set another and work towards that. Your journey won't seem so long with all these pit stops.

This approach worked for students at the Brooklyn College of the City University of New York who aimed to eat more fiber. Those who set short-term goals, such as boosting their fiber intake by 5 grams a week, ate 91 percent more fiber than the students who did not set goals.

Be reasonable. The key is to set realistic, reachable goals. If you try to lose 50 pounds by next Tuesday, you're going to be disappointed.

Remember, if you trim 10 percent from your body weight, you've completed a successful weight-loss program. But University of Pennsylvania researchers recently discovered that obese people often aim for weight losses two to three times greater than that. No wonder they often get discouraged and give up.

Successful weight loss is a marathon, not a sprint. Slow and steady wins the race.

Chew some fat. Face it — low-fat diets are no fun. The good news is you don't need to lose taste to lose waist.

A Harvard study found that people on a moderate-fat, Mediterranean diet fared better than people on a strict low-fat diet. Why? They had tastier food options. For example, they could sauté vegetables in a bit of olive oil rather than steam them or use nonfat cooking spray.

After 18 months, only 20 percent of the low-fat dieters were still on the program, while more than half of the moderate-fat eaters were still going strong. What's more, the Mediterranean group lost an average of 9 pounds, while the low-fat group actually gained 6 pounds.

The low-fat group limited their fat to 20 percent of their total calories, while the Mediterranean group upped it to 35 percent. Adding just a bit more fat might help you subtract more weight in the long run.

You can lose weight and keep it off. Just make a few changes in your diet, set reasonable, short-term goals, and keep your meals interesting. Sure beats eating nothing but grapefruit for weeks, doesn't it?

Simple tricks take off the pounds

Everybody is doing it. In a recent Gallup poll, six in 10 Americans admitted they have tried to lose weight. The key word is "tried." If you're dieting, you know how tough losing those love handles can be. The benefits are worth it, though — a longer life with fewer health problems.

Simply trying to lose weight saves lives, says the Centers for Disease Control. People who try in vain to drop pounds are still more likely to live than people who never even give it a go. Those who succeed reap big rewards, too.

▶ Slimming down is the single most effective way to lower your triglycerides, plus it ups your "good" HDL cholesterol and slashes "bad" LDL cholesterol.

▶ Shedding as few as five to 10 pounds may even drop your high blood pressure enough for you to stop taking medication.

▶ Trimming just a few calories a day could thwart age-related damage throughout your body and add years to your life. Being overweight, however, starts slowing your memory in middle age and may raise your risk of dementia.

Make the right things easy and the wrong things hard. As with everything, there is a good and a bad way to shape up. You can try to change your lifetime habits through willpower alone, but that's pretty difficult. Temptation is everywhere. Vowing to make changes

On the horizon — new way to curb cravings

When it comes to food cravings, a tiny area of the brain may be to blame. Scientists studying people who quit smoking with no effort think a change in the insula, a small area of the brain, may be at work. They looked at 19 former smokers with damage to their insula regions from surgery, stroke, or other causes.

Of these people, 18 later completely lost the urge to smoke. They didn't even have to try to quit. The insula controls your body's internal conditions and your conscious desires, like the urge to eat. Perhaps in the future, doctors can use this connection to help dieters kick their cravings for sweets, fast food, or milk shakes.

without thinking ahead to the pitfalls is setting yourself up for failure, as many dieters know. Instead, make things easy on yourself. Develop a plan with specific strategies to change your habits in small ways. For example, instead of dining out at an all-you-can-eat buffet, try a restaurant that offers smaller portions or tasty low-fat options. If you love cherry cheesecake, buy one slice but don't bring the whole cheesecake home.

Get to know your bathroom scale. You may be in the habit of weighing yourself every week, but that's not enough. Experts say a

Tangy fruit battles the bulge

The old-fashioned "grapefruit diet" may be just a fad, but including this citrus fruit in your weight-loss plan really works. Research shows eating grapefruit three times a day helps you curb your appetite and regulate your insulin. Overweight people who ate half a grapefruit before each meal lost an average of 3.6 pounds in a 12-week study. They also enjoyed small improvements in their insulin levels.

People in other test groups tried drinking grapefruit juice and taking capsules of dried grapefruit. These groups lost some weight, but not as much as the fruit eaters. Only the real fruit helped regulate insulin. Along with these benefits, experts say naringin, a flavonoid in grapefruit, slows absorption of fats and carbohydrates in your intestines.

A word of caution — drinking grapefruit juice can cause certain medications, like blood pressure drugs, to build up to toxic levels in your body. Ask your doctor or pharmacist if grapefruit juice will affect your medication.

daily weigh-in is best to keep you on track. A recent study of more than 3,000 people trying to either lose weight or keep weight off found better results for those who hopped on the scale every day. In fact, people trying to lose weight who weighed daily lost an average of twice as many pounds as those who stayed off the scale. Experts think frequent feedback — good or bad — may help you make small changes to move closer to your dieting goals. If you find the numbers on your scale moving slowly in the wrong direction, try small fixes like skipping desserts for a week or making time for an extra walk each evening.

Go for the slow burn. The best way to slim down and stay that way is to aim for a slow, steady rate of weight loss. The gradual change may not feel as rewarding as suddenly dropping a lot of pounds, but you're much more likely to stay slim and trim, and much less likely to suffer with gallstones and other side effects of rapid weight loss.

Be reasonable. Don't aim to lose more than 10 percent of your body weight, at least at first. You may be tempted to give up if the goal seems too hard to reach. Plus, cutting too many calories can actually slow your metabolism, making it tough to shed those pounds.

Try the buddy system. Enlist the aid of your spouse, partner, or best friend. Invite them to join your diet if they need to lose weight. Sticking to your guns — and your weight-loss plan — is easier with moral support and a sympathetic ear. Besides that, being on the same eating plan as your partner simplifies shopping and cooking, and you won't be tempted to poach naughty foods from another's plate.

Keep a diary. Use it to log your daily food and activities. Many studies show tracking your food and exercise habits will help you lose weight and keep it off. Also, note your weigh-ins. Seeing your progress in black and white will motivate you during the tough times, and you may discover patterns of eating and behavior that have kept you overweight all these years.

Milk your diet to burn fat

Americans are 25 pounds heavier than they were in 1960, according to the National Center for Health Statistics — but help may already be in your refrigerator. Some studies say you can raise your metabolism and drop pounds with the calcium in dairy products.

Scientists suspect calcium helps determine whether you burn fat. When your calcium levels sink too low, your body thinks you're starving, so it stores fat. When calcium is high, you burn fat more efficiently — and perhaps discard more fat in your waste, too. So you might rev up your metabolism and slim down with calcium.

Losing weight may even limit your ability to absorb calcium, according to a recent study of postmenopausal women. And that might mean older women need extra calcium when they're shedding pounds.

Just by adding creamy and delicious yogurt to your diet, you could score big — like the group in a Tennessee study who lost 61 percent more body fat than those who cut calories but didn't add in extra calcium.

Review the evidence. Two separate reviews examined the research on calcium and weight. Both found enough evidence to conclude that a high calcium intake may help prevent weight gain and may even purge some pounds — but scrimping on calcium might have the opposite effect.

What's more, both reviews agree that dairy calcium seems to have a bigger impact on weight loss than calcium from supplements. Experts think that other dairy ingredients might be pitching in to help.

Yet many clinical human studies have been too small, too short, or funded by the dairy industry. That's why large clinical trials and further research are still needed to help settle issues like how calcium affects weight, how safe and effective it may be, and the best way to use it. Because the jury is still out on the calcium-weight loss connection, the Federal Trade Commission recently ruled that dairy producers must stop claiming their products cause weight loss until research provides stronger evidence.

Become a clever calcium consumer. Still, adding more calcium is probably a good idea for most of us. After all, more than half of all adults in the U.S. don't get the recommended amount of calcium – which is 1,000 to 1,200 milligrams (mg) per day for older adults. Just adding one to two servings of dairy (from 300 to 600 mg of calcium) to your diet every day, could make a difference in your weight and your health.

While calcium might keep your metabolism from sabotaging your weight, this nutrient isn't a miracle pill. Calcium only helps you lose

Know your obesity risks

What is the difference between being overweight and being obese? You are overweight if you weigh more than the average person for your height. The extra weight can come from bone, muscle, or fat. Obesity is having a dangerously high proportion of body fat and is a risk factor for chronic conditions like diabetes and heart problems.

Who is more likely to gain extra weight? People who are sedentary, who eat more calories than they use, or those with a family history of obesity are more likely to carry too much weight.

Who is at greater risk for disease because of weight?

▶ men with a waist measurement greater than 40 inches

▶ women with a waist measurement greater than 35 inches

weight if you're already on a reduced-calorie diet. So add calcium-rich dairy to your meals only if you cut calories somewhere else — and favor dairy choices that are low in fat and calories.

Both dairy lovers and dairy haters can benefit from calcium. If you love dairy, try these easy ways to slip dairy foods into a low-calorie diet.

▶ Add low-fat milk to your coffee and tea.

▶ Enjoy a half cup of low-fat frozen yogurt.

▶ Don't be fooled by sour cream, cream cheese, coffee creamer, or whipped cream. They're all low-calcium wimps.

▶ Add two servings of low-fat yogurt to your daily menu. Mix in some fruit for a treat.

▶ Trade in that high-calorie milk shake for a smoothie blended with fruit, ice, and low-fat milk.

▶ Sprinkle fat-free dry milk powder on almost anything. You won't notice the taste or calories, and 2 tablespoons add about 100 mg of calcium.

If you hate dairy, get calcium from sources like canned sardines with bones, calcium-fortified orange juice, kale, and hearty fortified cereals. You can also try a daily dose of around 500 mg of calcium citrate.

Popular diets: what works, what doesn't

From diets featuring peanut butter and ice cream to those pushing grapefruit, there seems to be a weight-loss strategy for every taste. Before you jump on the latest bandwagon, see how your diet rates against this standard.

▶ For a diet to work, you must eat fewer calories than you burn.

▸ Your food choices should provide all the vitamins, minerals, and other nutrients you need to stay healthy.

▸ A successful diet will be diverse, so you never get bored and give up.

Here's how some of today's most popular diets stack up.

High-protein/low-carb diets. Eating plans similar to the Atkins diet recommend you cut carbohydrates without restricting fat or protein. Presumably, your body burns more fat when it isn't supplied with a steady stream of easy carbohydrates to burn. Recent short-term studies show some people lose more weight on this diet than on a low-fat diet. Surprisingly, this eating plan can also lower your cholesterol. But before you banish carbohydrates, remember your diet must provide all the nutrients you need. When you limit vegetables, fruit, and grains, you put your health at risk.

In addition, a high-protein diet usually means more saturated fat – which can block your arteries – along with an overabundance of ketones – waste products from protein and fat. A buildup of ketones in your blood, called ketosis, can increase your body's production of uric acid, a risk factor for gout and kidney stones. This condition is especially risky for people with diabetes. Until there are more long-term studies, get your doctor's approval and supervision before you begin this type of diet.

Low-fat diets. Eating plans like the Dean Ornish Life Choice Program stress an almost vegetarian lifestyle, with only 10 percent of your calories coming from fats. Ornish suggests that your body is designed to function best on a diet of mostly plant-based foods. It stores fat – or energy – for later, when you might need it. If you cut out fat and eat a varied diet of fruit, vegetables, whole grains, and beans, you will fill up faster and speed up your metabolism. Along with diet, Ornish also encourages you to exercise, manage stress, and stay connected to friends and family. He says you can not only lose weight, but also reverse the effects of heart disease with this diet and lifestyle.

Keep in mind this diet is strict. You might have a hard time cutting meat and fats (including olive oil) and avoiding sugar and salt. Getting enough fresh, unprocessed foods will undoubtedly be a challenge for many people in today's fast-paced society. You'll also need to watch your nutrient intake to make sure you don't become deficient in vitamins E, B12, and D, as well as calcium. However, if you eat a variety of vegetarian protein sources – like rice plus beans – you should meet your body's amino acid requirements.

Medium-fat diets. These diets loosely follow the eating habits of Mediterranean cultures – Greeks, southern French, and some Italians, for example – who usually get more than 30 percent of their calories from fat. But it's not just any fat – they eat "good" monounsaturated fat from olive oil and nuts, and they get less saturated fat. The Mediterranean diet also recommends fish, fruits, vegetables, and beans, along with using whole grains and yogurt freely.

This eating plan may be the perfect balance between the low-fat and high-protein diets. It's diverse and flavorful enough to keep you on the diet, but it cuts back on harmful fats and refined grains. It also lines up with official health organizations' recommendations for acceptable intakes of fat and carbohydrates.

Prepared meal plans. These programs deliver precooked balanced meals – usually low-fat and low-calorie – directly to your door. Research shows this approach can work, resulting in weight loss, improved heart health, and – perhaps most importantly – an improved quality of life.

Liquid and supplement diets. Replacing one to three meals a day with just a shake can be a hard regimen to stick to. But research shows if you're diligent, it can work – even over the long haul. This kind of diet seems especially beneficial to people who simply cannot change their eating habits. Controlling your food intake for even one meal is a daily reminder not to overeat.

Food points systems. Diets like Weight Watchers assign points to every food based on fat, fiber, and calorie content. You can pick and choose what you want to eat as long as you stay within a certain number of points every day. For motivation, you can join a weekly accountability group that keeps you on track. These diets can work as long as you don't cut out foods with good nutrients just because they have high point values.

Fad diets. Diets that promise fast and major weight loss often sound too good to be true. That's because they are. Be wary of any diet that is trying to sell a product, one based on testimonials instead of solid research, or one that excludes whole categories of food. Remember, too, that many natural or herbal weight-loss products are not reviewed or given approval by the U.S. Food and Drug Administration (FDA).

The FDA recommends you plan to lose just one to two pounds a week on any diet. Your best bet is to eat 300 to 500 fewer calories every day and exercise regularly — a winning recipe for steady, permanent weight loss.

Shop around for best diet help

There is plenty of help out there for people trying to lose weight. You can choose a plan that tells you what to eat, one that includes counseling, or even one that delivers food to your door. But be ready to pay the price for convenience.

Before you sign up with a plan, ask about what you'll get for your money. Weight Watchers, the Zone, and other commercial programs offer weight-loss tips and support groups to help you make lifestyle changes. Some programs, like Jenny Craig and Nutrisystem, also sell prepackaged meals. Nutrisystem offers a special plan for people with type 2 diabetes. These programs can be expensive, but they could help you reach your weight-loss goal. Take Off Pounds Sensibly (TOPS) is a nonprofit group and the least expensive of the programs. See the table on the following page for an overview of the different programs.

Weight-loss plan	Fees	Plan structure	Food	Support
Jenny Craig	$6 a week and up, plus cost of food	diet control with Jenny Craig prepackaged food	buy from Jenny Craig for $11–$15 a day	one-on-one counseling, either in person or by phone
Nutrisystem	cost of food only	diet control with Nutrisystem prepackaged food	buy from Nutrisystem for $289 a month	counseling, classes, newsletter, all at home or online
Take Off Pounds Sensibly (TOPS)	$24 a year plus nominal chapter fees	encouragement to stick with food and exercise plans from member's own doctor	buy and prepare your own	weekly chapter meetings, newsletter
The Zone	$52 every 13 weeks	meal planner, recipes, shopping lists	buy and prepare your own	daily tips, online nutritionists
Weight Watchers	$39.95 a month	instruction on eating plans for weight loss	buy and prepare your own	weekly meetings, lower fee for online plan

Win with old-fashioned calorie counting

When it comes to losing weight, calories are key. To lose weight, your body will have to use up more energy than it gets from food. Scientists measure food energy in calories. If you eat more calories than you use up during the day, you gain weight. If you burn off more calories than you eat, either by exercising more or simply eating less, you lose weight. Many current fad diets use this advice, then dress it up to make it more interesting to weary dieters.

Everyone needs a different number of calories to maintain weight or lose weight. A doctor could help you determine your specific needs, but here are some examples:

▶ If a 55-year-old woman who is 5 feet, 5 inches tall and weighs 135 pounds does four hours of very light activity, like reading or driving, and 30 minutes of light activity, like sweeping or walking, she would need 1,705 calories a day to maintain her current weight.

▶ If a 55-year-old man who is 5 feet, 10 inches tall and weighs 155 pounds does four hours of very light activity and 30 minutes of light activity, he would need 1,975 calories to maintain his current weight.

According to nutritionists, if you are an average-size person and you consistently eat about 1,400 to 1,500 calories a day, no matter how much physical activity you get, you will probably lose weight. You may need to adjust that number up or down a little if you are taller and more muscular or smaller than most. Dietitian Dawn Jackson, a spokesperson for the American Dietetic Association (ADA), says, "In general, we know a 1,500-calorie diet is good for weight loss, and you don't have to go much lower."

Losing weight is easier if you eat foods that make you feel full. You're also less likely to binge or snack constantly. Here's the low-down on foods, from most filling to least.

Bring on the boiled potatoes. According to a Satiety Index developed by Australian researchers, a boiled potato is the most satisfying and filling food you can eat. It also scores low on the glycemic index.

Hail those high-fiber foods. Fiber fills you up because it absorbs water and swells, taking up more space. Fiber also slows the movement of food through your upper digestive tract, so you don't get hungry as quickly. Good sources of high-fiber include fruits, vegetables, legumes, and grains such as oats, barley, wheat, rice, and rye.

Fill up without filling out

Trick your body into losing weight. Here's a strategy that melts off fat safely, naturally, and easily.

Studies show that people tend to eat the same amount of food, regardless of calories. So instead of trying to limit how much you eat, pay attention to your food's energy density. That means the number of calories in each gram. The more fiber or water in a food, for instance, the lower its energy (or calorie) density. You'll feel more satisfied after eating it — but you'll be getting fewer calories. For example, soups have a low energy density because of their high water content. Vegetables are less energy dense than, say pasta. Another trick is to beat foods. Add air by turning ice cream into a milkshake, and you'll be more satisfied with less.

These tricks could let you lose weight while eating as much — or more — than you do now.

Love those beans and lentils. Also high in fiber, beans and lentils make you feel full and leave you feeling full longer because your body absorbs them slowly.

Go the whole-grain way. When it comes to bread, whole grain is 50 percent more filling than white bread.

Snack on popcorn rather than Snickers. Popcorn will make you feel twice as full as a candy bar or peanuts will. Cakes, cookies, and donuts also measured up as some of the least-filling foods.

Favor fish over beef or chicken. Calorie for calorie, fish fills you up better than beef or chicken.

Opt for oranges and apples. When it comes to filling fruit, oranges and apples outscore bananas every time.

Pick porridge over cold cereal. It's almost always 50 percent more filling, and many times it's twice as filling.

Give croissants the cold shoulder. They're the least filling food of all.

When trying to decide between two foods of equal caloric value, go with the food that weighs more. Generally, researchers have found the heavier food to be the most filling. Another way to determine how filling a food is likely to be is to look it up in your calorie book, and compare the calories to the portion size. Limit foods that have more than 250 calories per 4-ounce portion.

Generally, carbohydrates make people feel fuller than any other food. Protein-rich foods, such as fish, meat, eggs, and cheese, come in second. But beware. If you're eating fewer than 1,500 calories a day, you're probably not getting all the nutrients your body needs. To keep yourself in tip-top shape, take a multivitamin/mineral supplement to be sure you're meeting your body's nutritional needs.

Keep yourself honest with a food diary

It's easy to say you're watching what you eat, but it's also easy to fool yourself. For successful weight loss, begin with awareness of what you really are eating – not what you think you are eating – by writing it all down.

Keep track of your calories. "Although people will always fight it, keeping a food diary improves self-awareness," says Dawn Jackson, Chicago dietitian and spokesperson for the American Dietetic Association. "We know from the National Weight Registry of thousands of people who have lost weight and kept it off, successful dieters monitor their food intake along with their weight."

You'll find a blank meal diary on the following page. Use it to log the foods you eat and the number of calories in each. You can use any reliable list of foods and their calorie contents to check your favorite foods. Write down every calorie – don't be tempted to fudge. You're the only one who needs to see this, and if it isn't accurate it won't be helpful.

Decide your daily calorie limit. After recording your calories for one week, add together your seven daily totals and divide that number by 7. This will give you the average calories you are eating each day.

No matter what the creators of fad diets say, the most important thing weight-loss champs know – and you should, too – is that to lose weight you must burn more calories than you take in. To lose one pound per week, you need to cut out 500 calories each day.

So, subtract 500 calories from your daily average, and you'll see how many calories you can eat a day and still meet your weight-loss goal.

Meal Diary (calculate how many calories you normally eat each day, then find your daily average)						
Sunday	**Monday**	**Tuesday**	**Wednesday**	**Thursday**	**Friday**	**Saturday**
Breakfast Calories:	Breakfast Calories:	Breakfast Calories:	Breakfast Calories:	Breakfast Calories:	Breakfast Calories:	Breakfast Calories:
Lunch Calories:	Lunch Calories:	Lunch Calories:	Lunch Calories:	Lunch Calories:	Lunch Calories:	Lunch Calories:
Dinner Calories:	Dinner Calories:	Dinner Calories:	Dinner Calories:	Dinner Calories:	Dinner Calories:	Dinner Calories:
Snack Calories:	Snack Calories:	Snack Calories:	Snack Calories:	Snack Calories:	Snack Calories:	Snack Calories:
Total						
Add up your daily totals to get your weekly total calories:						
Divide by 7						
Average daily calorie intake:						

Top tips for when the dieting gets tough

Your weight-loss plans are going smoothly. You're in the groove of your new eating plan, and your blood sugar is under control. At last, you even found an exercise class you enjoy with people you like, and you look forward to evening walks with your husband.

Then – boom. Something happens to upset the balance, and your diet is thrown off track. Maybe it's the start of the winter holiday season, or maybe your grandson's birthday party reminds you how much you miss eating ice cream and chocolate cake. Or perhaps you're invited to a church supper where everything but the sugar-sweetened iced tea is served batter-dipped and deep-fried. What can you do to stay on the weight-loss wagon?

They say if you fail to plan, you plan to fail. When it comes to losing weight, in other words, you need to think ahead about the difficulties that will block your path.

Determine your eating weaknesses. Everybody has them – those foods you just can't resist. The best way to manage those cravings is to allow small indulgences from time to time. Of course, it's best if your favorite treat also has some health benefit. Although an ounce of dark chocolate, for example, has about 150 calories, it may be good for your heart. If cookies are your weakness, consider those that are fruit-filled, like Fig Newtons. They provide lots of fiber and antioxidant nutrients.

If you're torn between a sweet beverage and a dessert, go for the solid. In one study, people who ate a sweet snack were less hungry and ate less at the next meal than those who drank a sugary drink with the same number of calories.

Recognize emotional eating triggers. Some people clean house when they are angry. Others can't seem to stop eating when they

Get fit with healthy habits

Eating right is only half your ticket to great looks and good health. Moving your body is the other half. Here are some easy ways to get your body in gear.

▸ Follow a European tradition and take a walk after dinner. Getting your body moving will get those digestive juices going.

▸ Thump your feet. Tap your fingers. Fidgeting is a form of exercise that can burn an average of 348 calories a day.

▸ Buy a pedometer and walk 10,000 steps a day.

▸ Ask about mall-walking programs near you.

▸ Learn new steps and meet new people at a dance class offered by your local recreation department.

▸ Make sleep a priority. Research indicates people snoozing fewer than six hours every night are more likely to be overweight.

are bored, sad, or lonely. To guard against binge eating at times of emotional stress, try these four steps.

▸ Figure out why the craving hits. Record in your food diary not only what you eat and how much, but also when, where, and what you are feeling. Knowing what events trigger eating sprees helps you prevent them.

▸ Think of things you could do instead of eating. Go for a walk or a bike ride, put on some music and dance out your frustrations, or call up a friend who will be a supportive listener.

▸ Give in occasionally. If you haven't allowed yourself a favorite comfort food lately – or at least a satisfying substitute – it may be harder to resist over-indulging when stress hits. Letting yourself savor a small dish of your favorite ice cream may be just what the doctor ordered for your mental and emotional health.

▶ Replace junk food with healthy choices. If you only have wholesome, low-calorie treats available, when the desire to binge hits, you won't do much damage. Keep a piece of fruit or a bag of baby carrots and other vegetable munchies handy, wherever you are.

Exercise to burn calories. You will drop some pounds by dropping calories, but if you want to keep the weight off, you have to exercise. You'll also reduce stress, which can contribute to weight gain. Exercise can also help you deal with a small slip from the dieting wagon by letting your body put these extra calories to good use.

Many experts believe walking is your best exercise choice. According to some studies, it may actually be more effective for trimming down than running or other popular physical activities. Because you are less prone to injury when walking, you are less likely to become an exercise dropout.

Rest well. At the end of a difficult day, you may wonder if you'll be able to hold to your new calorie goal. But after a good night's sleep, your confidence should bounce back. One study suggests that willpower returns after rest or a positive emotional experience.

Dine out with care. Don't avoid restaurants because you're trying to lose weight — just have a plan so that the menu doesn't sabotage your best intentions. These tips should help you enjoy the experience and stick to your calorie count.

▶ Opt for lunch. The portions are generally smaller than at dinner.

▶ Go light. Choose a restaurant with "light" dishes on the menu. Or call ahead to see if the chef will make adjustments, like grilling an item that's usually fried or substituting steamed vegetables for french fries.

Jump start your metabolism to burn fat fast

Eating breakfast helps you lose weight — and keep it off. Nearly four out of five people in the National Weight Control Registry, a survey of almost 3,000 people who have lost at least 30 pounds and kept it off for a year or more, eat breakfast every day. So don't rush out of the house in the morning before you fuel up for the day.

The right kind of breakfast keeps you from getting hungry and loading up on calories later in the day. Choose whole-grain cereals and fruit, but steer clear of sugary cereals. Sugar, a simple carbohydrate, raises your blood sugar quickly — then it falls, and you're hungry again. Both whole grains and eggs, another breakfast favorite, will help you feel full longer.

▸ Divide and conquer. Ask for a take-out container at the beginning rather than the end of a meal. Fill it with half your food — two-thirds if the restaurant serves extra-large portions — before you begin to eat. You can divide it again when you get home, then freeze or refrigerate it for later meals.

▸ Skip the entrees. Instead, make your meal from a salad, broth-based soup, and a low-calorie appetizer — like shrimp cocktail.

▸ Ban the buffet. If you can't avoid an all-you-can-eat food bar, limit yourself to two trips. Load up a dinner plate with fruits, salads, and other low-calorie vegetable dishes. If you eat it all and still want more, use a small salad plate for the second visit.

▸ Allow sensible treats. When a pizza craving hits, order a veggie special on thin crust with double tomato sauce and a light sprinkling of cheese.

Avoid holiday setbacks. If you have a clear plan, you're less likely to stumble on the path to a trimmer, healthier you during the holidays – when events and parties often revolve around eating. Have an emergency strategy. If you know that an upcoming holiday season is usually a "code red" – when your careful eating routine is bushwhacked – lower your expectations. Think ahead and go to a maintenance-level eating plan for those times when losing weight will temporarily be more difficult. To maintain your weight, plan to allow yourself more calories than while losing weight. Add about 100 more daily calories – but only until the holidays are over. Then climb back on the wagon.

Don't get discouraged if you do have a setback. Acknowledge it happened, put it behind you, and recommit to your plan. "Aim for progress and not perfection," says Dawn Jackson, Chicago dietitian and spokesperson for the American Dietetic Association.

Dissolve your calories with water

What a splash it would make if you could effectively lose weight by drinking lots of water. Some people are giving it a try and swearing by it. Although swimming is a time-tested weight-loss regimen, water may work its magic inside your body as well.

Know water's worth. Health and nutrition textbooks are a wellspring of information on the importance of water to your body. It transports nutrients, cleanses cells, carries away waste, lubricates joints, cushions organs, and regulates body temperature. Drinking eight to 10 glasses a day is a healthy habit, but will it also help you lose weight?

Some experts say drinking lots of water will make you feel full, so you'll be less likely to overeat. Others say water may help clear wastes from your body more efficiently. But research points to a possible effect on metabolism as the key to water's value in weight loss. Drinking a lot of water may actually raise your metabolic rate, which is the rate at which you burn calories. In one study, drinking

Delicious food sources of water	
Food	**Water content by weight**
1 head of iceberg lettuce	95 percent
1 large cucumber, unpeeled	95 percent
1 wedge of watermelon	91 percent
1 raw papaya	88 percent

cold water after a meal led to an increase in fat burning in men, while in women, drinking water increased carbohydrate burning.

Check out the research. One study by scientists in Germany and Canada looked at the influence of drinking water on metabolism. Their findings suggest water increases your metabolic rate within 10 minutes of drinking it and lasts for an hour or more. They found that drinking 1.5 liters (6 cups) of water each day could help you burn 48 more calories. That adds up to 17,400 calories per year or about 5 pounds.

Nevertheless, reviews of this research are mixed. Some suggest the study was too small, with only 14 people participating. Other critics claim the additional calories burned by drinking extra water won't necessarily translate into noticeable weight loss. Of course, if your daily water replaces high-calorie sodas and other beverages, that could be a different story.

Uncover clever sources of water. Don't overlook water "supplements" in your weight-loss program, either. Many tasty fresh fruits and vegetables are 80 to 99 percent water. Try cucumbers, lettuce, summer squash, watermelon, grapefruit, strawberries, apples, and tomatoes for the most water-dense additions to your diet.

The jury is still out on whether water truly has an impact on weight loss, but scientists agree it provides great benefits to your body, so it can't hurt to try. When it comes to managing your weight, every little health improvement can be significant.

Simple strategy to cut body fat

Permanent weight loss is hard. The conventional approach involves two basic principles:

▶ Eat a high-carbohydrate, low-fat diet with plenty of fruits, vegetables, and whole grains, while cutting down on meat and other sources of saturated fat.

▶ Burn more calories than you take in. In other words, eat less and exercise more.

Now there is another, slightly more controversial, strategy that has shown results for some people.

Drop pounds with protein. A high-protein diet, like the high-carbohydrate diet, limits fat to 30 percent of your daily calories. However, it doubles the amount of protein while reducing the amount of carbohydrates. You end up with a 40-30-30 carbohydrate-to-protein-to-fat ratio instead of the 55-15-30 percentage recommended by the USDA Food Guide Pyramid.

Dr. Donald K. Layman, a professor of foods and nutrition at the University of Illinois, conducted a small study that demonstrated the benefits of a higher protein diet. In the study, 24 overweight women ate a 1,700-calorie diet for 10 weeks. Half followed the recommendations of the USDA, while the other half ate the 40-30-30 diet. Both groups lost roughly the same amount of weight (about 16 pounds), but the higher protein group lost more fat and less muscle than the other group. They also lowered their triglycerides, or fat in the blood, and slightly raised their HDL (good) cholesterol.

"The protein diet was twice as effective," Dr. Layman said. "Women eating the lower protein diet were less capable of burning calories at the end of the study as when they started it. We believe this is the effect of more protein, particularly the increased amount of leucine in the diet." Leucine, an amino acid found in protein, is important for normal growth and metabolism. It also provides fuel for your muscles and helps maintain blood sugar after exercise.

Keep a grip on blood sugar. Of special interest to people with diabetes or those at risk for diabetes is protein's favorable effect on glucose, or blood sugar. Many carbohydrates, especially highly

7 sensible steps for long-term success

Weight-loss fads come and go. But common sense and a healthy plan of attack will help you melt off pounds — and keep them off.

▶ Drink water every day.

▶ Eat plenty of whole grains, legumes, and fresh fruits and vegetables.

▶ Cut back on sweets, refined carbohydrates, processed foods, and unhealthy fats.

▶ Get at least 30 minutes of moderate exercise every day.

▶ Keep a food diary, writing down everything you eat.

▶ Sit down to eat, concentrate on your food, and push the plate aside when you're full — whether it's empty or not.

▶ Rinse your mouth with a mixture of one teaspoon of baking soda dissolved in a glass of warm water. This folk remedy claims to turn off a craving for sweets. Be sure not to swallow the mixture.

refined carbohydrates, cause a major rise in blood sugar after a meal. Without enough insulin to properly handle the extra glucose, it is absorbed into the body as fat. Protein, on the other hand, doesn't cause this kind of rise. Some experts even recommend a bit of protein before bedtime to protect against bouts of nighttime hypoglycemia.

Know the perils of protein. While high-protein diets, like the Atkins diet, can lead to short-term weight loss, they come with some drawbacks.

▶ Most people find the diet boring and tough to stick to. Once you go back to eating a normal amount of carbohydrates, your weight comes back, too.

▶ With all that meat comes a lot of saturated fat, the kind that causes cholesterol build-up in your arteries. You may lose weight, but you may also increase your risk for heart disease, stroke, and cancer.

▶ A high-protein diet may affect how well your kidneys work and therefore would be dangerous for people with diabetes who have kidney problems.

▶ While you load up on steak, pork, eggs, and other usual dieting outlaws, you are severely limiting carbohydrates, including fruit, some vegetables, and bread. Your body must look elsewhere for energy. It first uses any carbohydrates you have stored, then it goes after stored protein from your muscles and organs, and finally it turns to stored fat.

As in any successful diet, this program tells you to also reduce total calories. Critics of high-protein diets say it's the reduced calories, not the additional protein, that's responsible for the weight loss. Most sources of health advice, including the American Diabetes Association, favor a balanced, high-carbohydrate, low-fat diet instead. The ADA recommends that no more than 10 to 20 percent of your calories come from protein. Be sure you talk to your doctor before increasing the protein in your diet.

How much protein is enough?

Here's an easy way to figure out your protein needs. If you're trying to lose weight, multiply your current weight by 10. That gives you the amount of calories you should eat each day. For example, a 160-pound person trying to lose weight should eat 1600 calories.

To find out the percentage of those calories that the American Diabetes Association says should come from protein, multiply the total calories by 15 percent, or .15. That's 240 calories. Because every gram of protein has 4 calories, divide this number by 4 to see how many grams of protein you need. When you divide 240 by 4, you get 60 grams of protein.

See the related list of high-protein foods below to see how your favorites stack up.

Protein power		
Here are a few examples of high-protein foods, including serving size and grams of protein.		
	Serving Size	**Protein**
Chicken breast, roasted, no skin	6 ounces	53 g
Tuna, canned, packed in oil	1 cup	42 g
Soybeans, dry roasted	1/2 cup	34 g
Ground beef patty, lean, broiled	4 ounces	32 g
Salmon, broiled or baked	4 ounces	31 g
Black walnuts, chopped	1 cup	31 g

13 ways to avoid restaurant pitfalls

Time is scarce for busy dieters, and sometimes it's just easier to let someone else do the cooking. Let's face it — it's almost impossible to dodge the drive-through window. But eating super-sized and deep-fried will play havoc with your diet. Here are 13 handy tips for the next time you dine out.

▶ Never, ever super-size a meal.

▶ Order a small or regular-size burger instead of the quarter-pounder with cheese. You'll cut 250 calories.

▶ Skip the large fries and save 540 calories. That's about the calorie equivalent of an entire healthy meal.

▶ Think grilled when choosing chicken or fish. Frying can cost you more than 100 calories.

▶ Call in a thin-crust veggie pizza. It's not only more nutritious, but it's also a calorie bargain. Compare its 190 calories per slice to the 470 calories you get from one slice of stuffed-crust meat-lover's pizza.

▶ Order the taco salad but don't eat that deep-fried taco shell. You'll shave 370 calories off your dinner tab.

▶ Ask for a separate take-out box as soon as you place your order. Then split your meal in half when you get it, and box it up for later.

▶ Choose your condiments wisely. Mustard has just 3 calories in one teaspoon, while mayonnaise has 19. And remember a teaspoon is not much — about the amount in one fast food condiment packet. Most people use much more.

▶ Green salads are great ways to fill your vitamin bank. But trade the croutons and Parmesan cheese for seeds, nuts, and vegetable toppings.

▶ Shun the creamy salad dressings and go for a vinaigrette. Ask for your dressing on the side, and use only half of it.

▶ Select vegetable sides instead of pasta salads at the buffet. Not only are they more nutritious, but they also can carry about 100 to 300 fewer calories.

▶ Stop after just one meat serving or calorie-laden side dish at the all-you-can-eat buffet. Try a bowl of soup instead.

▶ Order water with lemon instead of a regular carbonated drink. You won't even notice the 120 to 150 calories you save with every glass.

Crack the code of foreign foods

Ethnic restaurants can have baffling menus. To figure out which dishes won't add to your weight, look for these menu tip-offs.

▶ **Italian.** Stay away from alfredo, carbonara, parmigiana, and anything that's stuffed or fried. Choose entrées described as primavera, piccata, marinara, grilled, or thin crust.

▶ **Chinese.** Crispy, crunchy, sweet and sour, and fried dishes are all loaded with calories. Look for steamed dishes and those containing these words: jum, kow, and shu.

▶ **Mexican.** Fill up on fajitas, entrées with shredded meat, soft corn tortillas, salsa, rice, or black beans. Eat nachos, chimichangas, guacamole, and taco salad shells only rarely.

▶ **French.** Lovely as they are, limit entrées with these words: pâté, crème, au gratin, fromage, hollandaise, en croûte, béarnaise, mousse, foie gras, or pastry. Instead, enjoy the delicate flavor of fruit sauces and choose poached, roasted, or en papillote dishes.

▶ **Indian, Thai, and Island fare.** Limit the amount of fritters and coconut dishes, and indulge in marinated, steamed, stir-fried, tandoori, tikka, and satay dishes.

Control your life to control your weight

The average American older than age 55 has added nearly 40 pounds of fat during adulthood. Much of the blame for this ugly fact goes to poor eating habits. Without making a few lifestyle changes, you'll always have a hard time maintaining a healthy weight. Here are some tips to help put you back in charge of your weight.

Practice portion control. Researchers at Cornell University discovered something interesting while hosting an ice cream social. When people serve themselves, they tend to put more food on their plates if the plates and serving utensils are large. Think small and cut back on the size of your helpings by using smaller plates, bowls, and serving utensils. When you're eating out, don't fall for the fast-food "supersize" craze. Cheap food that makes you gain weight is no bargain.

Fight hunger with brown rice

This nutty-tasting whole grain supplies healthy fiber to fill you up. But that's not all. New research may have found a way to learn how to control the "hunger hormone" and crush cravings for good. A small study suggests that hunger-boosting changes in the levels of two hormones that influence hunger could be linked to lack of sleep.

More research will determine whether sleep loss affects how ravenous you get. But why not try some steaming brown rice an hour or so before bed? This grain has melatonin, a natural hormone that helps regulate your body's daily rhythms and promotes sleep. Other foods with the highest levels of melatonin include oats, rice, corn, bananas, tomatoes, and cherries.

Pound the pillow. Women who sleep only five or six hours a night gain more weight than those who get seven hours of sleep a night, according to the Nurses' Health Study. Another study found that two key hormones that regulate appetite get out of whack when you don't get enough sleep. Leptin, which tells your body you've eaten enough, decreases, and ghrelin, which stimulates your appetite, increases.

Turn off the TV. Your risk for obesity increases 23 percent for every two hours a day you spend in front of your TV. Americans now burn 111 fewer calories a day than they did in years past, and that adds up to 11 pounds a year. When you're sitting around watching TV, not only does your metabolism slow, but you might be tempted by clever advertisers to reach for high-sugar, high-fat snacks – and empty calories.

Volunteer your services. Retirees who joined a program to help mentor and tutor children in local elementary schools more than doubled their physical activity, a Johns Hopkins University survey shows. Not only did the volunteers get off the couch and away from the TV, they had more energy for daily activities like household chores and gardening.

Find strength in numbers. You can lose more weight by joining an organized weight-loss group than if you try to go it alone, says a study funded by the U.S. Department of Agriculture. Women dieting on their own have higher stress levels, and that leads to less success overall. A group also gives you support and nutritional information you won't get by yourself.

Don't use food as a crutch. When you eat to cope with anger, depression, or stress, you're loading up on food that makes you fat. Find something else to help you deal with your emotions – go for a walk, take a relaxing bath, or play a game.

Forget about skipping meals. Eating three meals a day and a healthful snack or two keeps your blood sugar stable and your hunger pangs under control. In addition, missing a meal can encourage you to overeat at the next meal. Overeating stretches your stomach, which continues to signal hunger until it gets back to normal size.

Get the skinny on diet pills

Americans spend $2 billion a year on diet pills of one kind or another. Do they work? Sometimes — but only when you also adopt lifestyle changes, like cutting calories and exercising more. What the pills won't do is magically melt pounds away while you sit on your couch and eat whatever you want.

Your doctor may prescribe one of several drugs to either curb your appetite or prevent your body from absorbing some of the fat you eat. Most of these weight-loss drugs are only approved for short-term use, and they all have unpleasant side effects. Some side effects are mild, like headaches or stomach cramps, but others are serious, like high blood pressure.

Here's something else to consider. Most weight-loss drugs lose their effectiveness over time, and some can become addictive or trigger depression. These drugs don't work the same for everyone, so the exact dosage and results vary. Weight-loss drugs can be put into three general categories:

Appetite suppressants. These include the many herbs, drugs, and supplements sold to either curb your appetite or make you feel full. Phentermine — the "phen" part of the discontinued diet drug Fen-phen — is the most common prescription appetite suppressant. Brand names, including Adipex, Ionamin, and Fastin, can cost two or more times as much as generic phentermine. Fen-phen was banned several years ago because fenfluramine, the "fen" ingredient, was linked to heart valve problems. Phentermine is not associated with heart problems.

Other prescription appetite suppressants include sibutramine (Meridia) and diethylpropion (Tenuate). Rimonabant (Acomplia) is sold in Europe and was under review by the U.S. Food and Drug Administration until it was withdrawn by the manufacturer.

Fat absorption inhibitors. These drugs reduce your body's absorption of some of the fat you eat. They come with unpleasant side effects, like gas and diarrhea. They also interfere with absorption of the fat-soluble vitamins A, D, and E, and other important nutrients. The only FDA-approved fat absorption inhibitor is orlistat (Xenical). It's also available in a weaker, over-the-counter version called Alli.

Metabolism boosters. This approach to weight loss, known as thermogenic therapy, suggests that certain natural compounds, like chromium, coenzyme Q10, and pyruvate, encourage your liver to increase energy in your cells and raise metabolism. These compounds are part of a host of unregulated diet remedies, which also includes appetite suppressants not approved by the FDA. They all have numerous side effects — many of them serious.

Experts say the best — and safest — way to lose weight and keep it off is to eat less and exercise more. Over-the-counter pills and so-called natural remedies are expensive, and they can cause dangerous side

Weight-loss 'supplement' your body needs

It's free. It's available to absolutely everybody. And it's essential to every weight-loss program. What is it? Exercise, of course. Without exercise, even the best weight-loss plan won't give you the results you're hoping for. As an added bonus, exercise helps you lose weight faster and keep it off longer. It's best to exercise at your target heart rate for 20 minutes with a 10-minute warm-up and a 10-minute cool-down. To find your target heart rate, subtract your age from 220 and multiply the result by 0.6.

effects. Plus, their reactions with other drugs are unknown. You need to be especially careful if you have a condition like diabetes. Never take a supplement without talking to your doctor first.

Diuretics: fast track to a heart attack

Taking diet pills may seem like a faster track to a slimmer figure than counting calories and exercising. But these medications can be dangerous, especially if you have heart problems, diabetes, or certain other diseases.

By the same token, don't be tempted to use diuretics, or water pills, to lose weight. They can disturb your body's electrolyte balance and put you at risk of a heart attack. They are especially dangerous when combined with a low-protein diet, which can starve your heart muscle and disturb heart rhythms.

Using water pills when taking other medicines is also risky business. "People taking diuretics are particularly vulnerable to dehydration," says cardiologist Dr. David Calhoun, director of the University of Alabama Birmingham Hypertension Clinic.

"The combination of depleted fluid volume and medication," he warns, "can lead to problems such as dangerously low blood pressure, particularly for older patients who are sensitive to becoming dehydrated."

If you take medications, Calhoun says to be sure to drink at least the recommended six glasses of water each day — more when you exercise or spend a lot of time in the sun.

Startling secret to weight loss

A hidden cause of weight gain may make dropping 25 pounds as easy as giving up your favorite vegetables.

Top 10 tips for easy weight loss

Try these fun and easy ways to lose weight permanently while you lower your blood pressure.

▸ Set realistic goals. Expect to lose 10 percent of your weight.

▸ Keep a food diary.

▸ Create a weekly food plan and leave room for the occasional treat.

▸ Cook your own meals to control your portion size, fat content, and nutrients.

▸ Eat five small meals a day. This may keep you from unhealthy snacks.

▸ Start your day with fiber-rich whole grains and fruit.

▸ Drizzle a little olive oil on your greens.

▸ Drink orange juice a half-hour to hour before each meal. This nutrient-loaded beverage helps you eat fewer calories.

▸ Sit down and savor your food. Stop eating when you feel full.

▸ Turn up the lights. You may be less likely to overeat if you can see your food.

So says Dr. Rudy Rivera, who maintains food intolerances are to blame for many of the weight problems people suffer. In his book, *Your Hidden Food Allergies Are Making You Fat,* co-authored with Roger D. Deutsch, Rivera tells of his own struggle with being overweight. Once he identified his food culprits — among them, carrots, broccoli, and green beans – he finally slimmed down and felt healthy.

True food allergies cause immediate reactions such as hives or wheezing, and they can be life-threatening. But when you're sensitive to a certain food, the reaction is not as obvious, Rivera says. It might not appear until hours or days later, and by then you wouldn't think of connecting the reaction to something you ate. Even so, an allergic-type reaction is invading your body. Your white blood cells can swell and burst, irritating the other cells. The result? You may feel exhausted, have a migraine, or keep gaining weight.

Rivera believes many cases of obesity are linked to this food-sensitivity cycle. He explains that, after your body reacts to an offending food, it becomes low in serotonin – a feel-good chemical that has a calming effect on your brain. Because eating carbohydrates can raise serotonin levels, you find yourself craving things like sugary snacks. Even worse, you'll probably crave the very foods you're sensitive to.

But you can break the cycle by figuring out which foods your body can't process. You can try eliminating foods from your diet one at a time to see if you notice any improvement, but this method can be difficult if you're sensitive to several foods. Rivera recommends the ALCAT test, a blood test for food intolerances. Along with identifying your problem foods, it tests for sensitivity to molds, chemicals such as preservatives, and food dyes. Rivera says once he stopped eating his trigger foods, he easily lost 25 pounds in a couple of months. But you have to stay away from your problem foods for at least three months, he says. After that, you can eat small amounts of the food again, but only occasionally. To avoid reactions, you should rotate foods so you never eat any food more than once every four days, he notes.

Your insurance company should pay for the ALCAT test if your doctor orders it, but check first. Some experts believe these types of allergy tests are not effective. If your doctor won't order the test, the company that designed it can refer you to another doctor, or you can do it at home. For more information, go to the Web site *www.alcat.com* or contact the American Medical Testing Laboratories Corp.: AMTL Corp., One Oakwood Blvd., Suite 130, Hollywood, FL 33020, 800-881-2685.

Learn food label lingo

Food labels can be confusing or even misleading. To help you out, the government has established definitions for terms used on food labels. Know what these terms mean so you know what you're getting.

- **Serving size.** The size may be much smaller or much larger than what you consider a single serving. Remember this when reading any per-serving figures.

- **Fat-free.** Less than 0.5 grams (g) of fat per serving.

- **Sugar-free.** Less than 0.5 g of sugar per serving. The term "low sugar" isn't regulated and may or may not mean what you expect.

- **Low-fat.** No more than 3 grams of fat per serving.

- **Good source of calcium.** At least 100 milligrams (mg) of calcium per serving. A good source of a nutrient must have 10 to 19 percent of the recommended daily value. An excellent source must have at least 20 percent.

- **Reduced.** At least 25 percent less fat, saturated fat, sodium, cholesterol, sugar, or calories per serving than the regular food.

- **Light or lite.** One-third fewer calories or half the fat of the higher-calorie, higher-fat food. Or half the sodium of a low-calorie, low-fat food.

- **Lean.** Less than 10 g of fat, 4 g of saturated fat, and 95 milligrams (mg) of cholesterol per serving of fish, poultry, or meat.

Drink from the fountain of youth

When you've successfully reached your weight-loss goal, your next objective might be to live to the ripe old age of 100 years. Dr. Roy Walford, author of *The Anti-Aging Plan* and *Beyond the 120-Year Diet*, thinks that's a reasonable notion.

Walford believes to extend your potential life span – the number of years you are likely to live – you must deeply and permanently reduce your calories. To stay healthy and mentally sharp throughout your longer life, all those calories should be jam-packed with nutrition.

Follow his anti-aging diet, Walford says, and you can substantially reduce your risk of most diseases that usually plague your middle and late years. His plan calls for gradual weight loss over six months to about a year. Then if you eat correctly, you can maintain your new "weight point" with your body operating at top efficiency and health.

Walford's books provide menus, recipes, and strict advice about working with your doctor.

Weigh the benefits of green tea

Green tea has been used for thousands of years to treat a variety of ailments. Today, this popular beverage is known for fighting cancer along with heart and respiratory disease, and many people claim its fat-fighting properties make it a natural complement to any healthy weight-loss program.

Know your teas. Green tea comes from the same plant as black and oolong teas. They're just processed differently. Those who love the full-bodied taste of black and oolong teas may be tempted to think green is too weak. But "weak" probably isn't the right word. Green tea is loaded with potent phytochemicals and antioxidants.

Steer clear of trendy 'diet' drink

Enviga, an expensive soft drink that contains green tea extracts, calcium, and caffeine, claims to burn 60 to 100 extra calories if you drink three cans in 24 hours. Unfortunately, the study that showed these benefits was based on healthy, normal-weight people ages 18 to 35.

Some studies suggest the antioxidants in green tea, called catechin polyphenols, might help with weight loss by restricting the activity of amylase, an enzyme in saliva that digests carbohydrates. Researchers think this action may slow the digestion of carbohydrates, which prevents the sudden rise of insulin in the blood and makes you burn fat instead of storing it. Others suggest the polyphenols in green tea increase your metabolism, helping you burn extra calories.

Try extract for biggest punch. In 1985, French researchers conducted one of the first trials on green tea's effect on fat. The study involved 60 middle-age, obese women who were put on a diet of 1,800 calories a day and took green tea extract at each meal for 30 days.

After two weeks, the green tea group lost twice as much weight as those on the same diet who took a placebo instead. After four weeks, the green tea group had lost three times as much weight as the placebo group − not to mention significantly greater losses in waist size.

More studies have been done since 1985, but most have focused on how many calories green tea extract burns, which doesn't always mean the same thing as losing weight.

The National Institutes of Health sponsored one of the most recent studies. In this study, 70 moderately obese adults took two capsules of green tea extract twice a day, containing a daily total of 375 milligrams of catechin.

After three months, their body weight dropped 4.6 percent (that's almost 10 pounds if you began at 200 pounds) and they lost 4.48 percent from their waist (2.25 inches if you began at 50 inches).

But here's the catch. You can melt pounds away with green tea, but not by drinking it. You would have to drink an awful lot of green tea to get the dose of fat-burning ingredients the participants in these trials received. They weren't drinking green tea. They were getting large doses of its active ingredients in green tea extract capsules.

Drink to good health. There's no question about it. Green tea's health benefits are amazing. But its usefulness as an aid to weight loss is clearly complementary – it helps. It complements a nutritious diet with limited portions and a daily exercise plan. So don't put your hopes for a dramatic drop in weight in green tea alone.

One more caution – unless the green tea you use is clearly marked "decaffeinated," it will contain caffeine. Although green tea has less caffeine than black tea and about one-third as much as coffee, too much might keep you awake at night or make you feel nervous. If this is true for you, switch to decaffeinated green tea. You can also buy decaffeinated green tea extract.

Maximize your weight-loss strategy

Chances are you need to add more fiber to your diet – especially if you want to lose weight. The average American eats only about 17 grams of fiber per day. That's around half the recommended amount. But the fact is, fiber is plentiful in healthy fruits, vegetables, and grains, and you can eat as much of it as your body can handle.

When the VA Medical Center in Lexington, Ky., compared eight diets – including the popular Atkins and Zone diets – they declared low-fat, high-fiber eating plans the healthiest. If you're trying to lose weight, fiber-rich foods will soon become your new best friends.

Get to know fiber. Fiber is divided into two main types – soluble and insoluble. Soluble fiber dissolves in water and becomes sticky in your digestive system. This characteristic slows down glucose absorption and helps lower cholesterol. That's good news for people with diabetes. Insoluble fiber doesn't digest. It moves quickly

Cereals – fiber heroes and fiber zeroes

Fiber heroes	Grams of fiber per serving
Kellogg's All-bran original	8.8
Wheatena (cooked with water)	6.6
Kellogg's Raisin Bran	7.3
Kellogg's Frosted Mini-Wheats bite-size	5.5
General Mills Raisin Nut Bran	5.1
General Mills Total Raisin Bran	5.0

Fiber zeroes	Grams of fiber per serving
Kellogg's Corn Flakes	0.7
General Mills Rice Chex	0.3
General Mills Honey Nut Chex	0.3
Kellogg's Corn Pops	0.2
Kellogg's Rice Krispies	0.1
General Mills Reese's Puffs	0.0

through your intestines, helping to keep you regular. Here's the secret to naturally block out calories from foods — just add fiber to your diet and watch the weight melt away.

▶ When fiber passes through your body without being digested, it provides little to no calories. Choosing fiber-rich foods instead of fats or sweets can make a big difference in your calorie intake.

▶ According to the USDA, increasing fiber decreases the digestibility of protein and fat so you end up absorbing fewer calories from these sources.

▶ Fiber also absorbs water and swells, making you feel full. Soluble fiber even slows the movement of food through your upper digestive tract, so you feel full longer. This means you're less likely to snack between meals.

Enjoy great results. The evidence for fiber as a weight-loss aid is overwhelming. Harvard researchers conducted one of the largest and longest studies. They tracked close to 75,000 healthy, middle-age women for 12 years and found those who ate the most high-fiber, whole-grain foods gained less weight than those who ate the most refined grains. In addition, the women who increased their intake of fiber or whole grains the most were half as likely to become obese over the 12-year period.

Set a fiber goal. The American Dietetic Association says people over age 50 should get 20 to 30 grams of both kinds of fiber per day. Younger people need 25 to 35 grams. Some experts recommend even more for your body to function at its peak. The bottom line is, you need to set a daily fiber goal. Experts have found that people with a target amount in mind are more likely to reach it than those who vaguely aim to increase their fiber intake.

But be careful. Adding too much fiber to your diet too quickly can lead to uncomfortable bloating and gas. Start slowly and drink lots of fluids.

The first meal of the day provides plenty of ways to get high-fiber foods, like fruit and whole-grain cereal, into your diet. In fact, Michigan State researchers found that women who ate cereal had significantly lower Body Mass Indexes (BMI) — perhaps because they ate less fat and more fiber. So if you want to lose weight fast, don't forget to eat a healthy breakfast.

Good sources of fiber include fruits and vegetables — especially with their skin — whole grains, beans, peas, seeds, wheat bran, oat bran, oats, barley, rye, and brown rice. You can also take fiber supplements, like Metamucil, for an added boost.

8 secret fiber-rich foods

Looking for a way to sneak more fiber into your meals? Try these simple, inexpensive, and tasty foods.

▶ Flaxseed. This tiny, nutritious seed may be the top weight-loss food. What's more, it protects your heart, eases arthritis, battles diabetes, and boosts your immune system. Grind flaxseed for best absorption, then sprinkle it on cereals or salads, bake it in breads, and stir it into sauces and stews.

▶ Potatoes. Boil or bake them in their skins. Leave off the butter, and instead top them with salsa or fat-free sour cream and chives. One medium potato has about 160 calories and 4 grams of fiber.

▶ Beans. Bake some great northerns or cook a pot of lentils. It takes a long time for your body to absorb these high-fiber foods, so you'll feel full longer.

▶ Whole-grain bread. Whole-wheat bread, for example, is much tastier, nutritious, and filling than white bread.

▶ Popcorn. Don't reach for a candy bar when this healthy low-calorie snack fills you up and keeps you satisfied longer.

▶ Apples. Munch on an unpeeled McIntosh — or another favorite — for a tasty alternative to low-fiber snacks.

▶ Oranges. They fill you up more than bananas, and the whole fruit provides more fiber than orange juice.

▶ Brown rice. This unprocessed grain gives you far more fiber than you'll find in white rice or pasta. High-fiber foods also help prevent constipation. It's important, however, to drink lots of water with them. Otherwise, they may have the opposite effect.

The only eating plan you'll ever need

There is only one eating plan that helps you drop pounds and keep them off for a lifetime. Here are the four most important rules of this successful plan:

Eat only what you can burn. Follow this advice and you may not have to worry about being overweight again. This is a "nothing forbidden" eating plan anybody can follow. What it means is, you can have that slice of cheesecake, but you have to burn those extra calories so your body won't store them as fat.

Once you get to your ideal weight, the only way to maintain it is to eat only as many calories as your body will burn in a day — 1,800 to 2,000 calories is about average.

Redistribute your calories. How you spend each day's allotment of calories is extremely important. The National Academy's Institute of Medicine (IOM) has set new guidelines for a balanced diet that are flexible and easy to follow. Because this healthy diet isn't as low on fat as you might think, you should be able to enjoy all your favorite foods — as long as you eat them in moderation. According to the IOM, divide your calories along these lines:

▶ 45 – 65 percent of calories should come from carbohydrates, the main component of grains, fruits, and vegetables.

▶ 20 – 35 percent can come from fat. But keep your intake of saturated fats as low as possible.

▶ 10 – 35 percent of your calories should come from protein sources, like meat, legumes, nuts, eggs, and dairy.

Most people find it hard to recognize the right proportion of protein to carbohydrates. The answer, however, is right before your eyes.

Get control of your portions. The American Institute of Cancer Research (AICR) recently published *The New American Plate*, which says eating right is all about portion and proportion. They explain an easy way to judge how much food is too much.

Take a look at your plate next time you sit down to dinner. If you eat like most people eat, meat might fill more than half your plate.

Sample serving sizes from the USDA

Item	Serving size	Compare to
whole vegetables and fruit	one medium vegetable or piece of fruit	a baseball
chopped vegetables and fruit	1/2 cup	a rounded handful
meat	3 ounces	a deck of cards
rice, mashed potatoes, or pasta	1/2 cup cooked	a tennis ball
snacks (nuts or pretzels)	1/3 cup	a level handful
cheese	1½ to 2 ounces	4 dice

According to Melanie Polk, R.D., Director of Nutrition Education at the AICR, this habit needs to change.

"Reverse the traditional American plate, and think of meat as a side dish or condiment rather than the main ingredient," Polk says. "Meat should only cover one-third or less of your plate."

"Plant-based foods," Polk says, "like vegetables, fruits, whole grains, and beans should cover two-thirds or more of your plate."

One way to switch to the new, healthier plate is to eat only half your usual portion of meat and have two vegetable sides instead of one. It's that simple.

Polk also notes that American serving sizes are far too big. In fact, obesity rates started climbing when restaurant portions tripled.

If you can't remember what a healthy portion should look like, there's an easy way to figure it out.

▸ Pull out two clean plates. On one, spoon out your usual portion of a food – for example, half a plate of noodles.

▸ Check the nutrition facts on the box of noodles and you'll discover that a serving size is probably around half a cup.

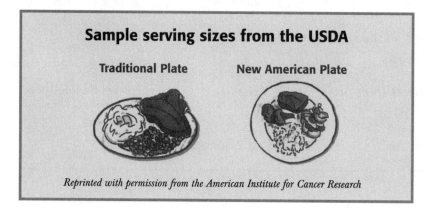

Sample serving sizes from the USDA

Traditional Plate   New American Plate

Reprinted with permission from the American Institute for Cancer Research

▶ Now measure out half a cup – or one serving – of noodles and place it on the second clean plate.

You might be surprised how small a single serving should be. "What we are recommending," says Polk, "is that if you weigh more than you would like to, or more than you should, take a look at your portion sizes and see how many standard serving sizes are included in those portions. Then start to cut down a little bit. This doesn't mean you have to cut out the food, it just means you may want to decrease the size of your portion."

Work your body. The crowning jewel of any healthy diet is exercise. The IOM recommends you exercise moderately for an hour every day. That's double the amount previously recommended by many experts. But exercise doesn't have to be done on a treadmill – you can climb stairs, take a walk, or do water aerobics. Even working hard at your chores counts as exercise.

Get a handle on challenging cravings

You have great intentions when it comes to watching what you eat, but sometimes double-fudge chocolate cake gets the best of you. Or maybe the prime rib special at your favorite eatery causes you to leap from the dieting wagon. Whatever your most challenging temptation is, you can learn to control the cravings. But you'll need to build up the mental muscles required for better self-control. Here's how to follow through on your good resolutions.

Don't expect perfection. While you're trying to develop healthy eating habits, don't expect to be perfect in other areas of your life. If you're feeling stressed about speaking in front of a crowd or dealing with a difficult relative, you may have trouble keeping to a low-calorie regimen. Stress in one area of life can weaken your resolve in other areas. Try to focus on one challenging task at a time to give yourself more chance for success.

Rate your weight

The body mass index (BMI) chart will help you decide if your weight is in a healthy range. A BMI of 25 or below is considered healthy. A BMI above 25 generally means you are overweight and above 30 indicates you are obese.

Weight (in pounds)	130	140	150	160	170	180	190	200
Height								
5'0"	25	27	29	31	33	35	37	39
5'1"	25	26	28	30	32	34	36	38
5'2"	24	26	27	29	31	33	35	37
5'3"	23	25	27	28	30	32	34	35
5'4"	22	24	26	27	29	31	33	34
5'5"	22	23	25	27	28	30	32	33
5'6"	21	23	24	26	27	29	31	32
5'7"	20	22	23	25	27	28	30	31
5'8"	20	21	23	24	26	27	29	30
5'9"	19	21	22	24	25	27	28	30
5'10"	19	20	22	23	24	26	27	29
5'11"	18	20	21	22	24	25	26	28
6'0"	18	19	20	22	23	24	26	27
6'1"	17	18	20	21	22	24	25	26
6'2"	17	18	19	21	22	23	24	26
6'3"	16	17	19	20	21	22	24	25

Look for help. If losing weight were easy, everyone would be successful the first time they tried. But it's not easy. Temptation is everywhere, and sometimes you may need help saying no. Avoid situations where you know you'll have trouble. For example, rather than a trip to the ice cream parlor, where temptation lurks, take your grandson to a playground. You'll both have fun with no willpower required. If you need more structure in your diet than you can create for yourself, join a dieting group like Weight Watchers or *www.eDiets.com*. There's strength in numbers.

Build self-control in other areas. Some psychologists promise if you flex the muscles of self-control in one area of your life, you'll have better results in other areas. Success in small attempts at willpower, like consistently avoiding a favorite after-work snack, can carry over into long-term dieting success. Try these baby steps.

▶ Practice sitting up straight, even if you must keep reminding yourself to do it.

▶ Brush your teeth with your less-dominant hand.

▶ Break the habit of saying "um" or "ah" as you speak.

Fool yourself into eating less

Drop pounds without dieting or even consciously watching what you eat. You can actually trick yourself into eating less by making small portions of food look bigger.

Years of study show it's not how much you eat that makes you feel full but how much you think you have eaten. By fooling your eyes into seeing portions as larger than they actually are, you can fool your stomach into feeling full with less food. Experts say trimming just 15 to 20 percent of your daily calories this way could help you lose 30 pounds in a year without trying.

Downsize your dishes. Use smaller plates and bowls at home. Bigger dishes create an optical illusion, so a normal-size scoop of food that fills a small plate looks lost on a big one. If a portion looks too small to your eyes, your stomach assumes it is, prompting you to eat more.

Even food experts fall for it. In one sneaky study, nutrition experts ate 30 percent more ice cream when they scooped it into extra-large bowls than they did using regular-size bowls. Similarly, when you serve yourself from a huge bowl or platter, you tend to take and eat more food than usual. Try substituting salad plates for your regular plates and serving meals from smaller platters and bowls.

Shrink your spoons. The size of your utensils matters, too. The ice cream–eating researchers dished up almost 15 percent more when they used large scoops compared to small ones. In another study, people were allowed to serve themselves as many M&M candies as they wanted. Halfway through the study, researchers swapped the small serving spoon in the bowl with a large one. People who used the big spoon ate twice as much candy as those who used the small spoon. So while trading in your big dishes, hunt

Eat deliberately

Writer Henry David Thoreau wanted to "live deliberately," to appreciate the events of each day. Do the same thing where food is concerned. Don't make a habit of eating while you watch television, talk on the phone, read the newspaper, or drive. Instead, pay attention to what you are eating and how much you consume. Trying to multi-task — eating while you do something else — makes it easy to lose track of how much you've eaten. That leads to overindulging. So make eating its own activity, and enjoy what you put in your mouth.

for smaller silverware, too, and make a point of serving meals with smaller spoons, scoops, and forks.

Go skinny with tall glasses. Drink high-calorie beverages, like soda and alcohol, from tall, slim glasses rather than short, wide ones, and you will automatically drink about 30 percent less. Short, wide glasses look like they hold less, so you tend to pour more into them than you think.

Plump up your food. The way you prepare the food you eat can trick your stomach just as surely as the size plates you use. People who normally ate a half-pound hamburger were given a quarter-pound burger dressed up with lots of lettuce, onion, and tomatoes to make it look as big as the half-pound burger. These hungry people felt just as full after eating the smaller burger as they did after eating the big one, but they consumed many fewer calories. Whipping air into foods to make them fuller and thicker has the same stomach-fooling effect.

Handy way to manage a hunger attack

Meals packaged like candy bars or milkshakes are tasty and convenient, but do they really help you lose weight? Some researchers think so. Although they'll never be a match for nutritious meals, they might be worth a try.

Zoom in on the facts. Eating a meal-replacement product, either in liquid or solid form, is a popular way to cut calories and lose weight. Many food bars are geared toward people on a particular weight-loss plan. They do offer certain advantages, like giving you a specific portion size and providing a convenient way to eat if you would skip a meal otherwise. This might help keep you from getting too hungry and overeating later. A recent study found certain meal-replacement products reduced hunger and the desire to eat for five hours after people ate or drank them.

Master midlife weight gain

You're not destined to jump three dress sizes just because you're going through menopause. With a little work, you can hold the scales steady. Most women gain an average of one pound per year during menopause. But by cutting calories, avoiding saturated fat, and exercising in your spare time, you can keep from gaining weight. In fact, you may actually drop a few pounds.

While weight control is important, other equally valuable health benefits can come from these lifestyle changes. You'll lower your blood pressure and help control insulin, cholesterol, and triglyceride levels.

Think of healthy eating and exercising as a way of pampering yourself through menopause and beyond. For moral support, join other women who have similar goals. Look for an aerobics or dance class, a swimming group, or a walking club.

Those who promote certain diet plans also claim that when you eat low- or moderate-carbohydrate foods, the insulin level in your blood won't rise as much after meals. This change may help you burn more fat and lose weight. However, studies have found these bars don't reduce insulin levels as much as expected.

Keep a close watch on blood sugar. People with diabetes know they shouldn't skip meals. Doing so can allow your blood sugar to drop to an unsafe level. But with your doctor's help, you may benefit from using certain meal-replacement bars or shakes to help lose weight. You may need to adjust your drugs to account for changing blood sugar levels when you begin to use meal replacements. Monitor your blood sugar carefully.

Take note of good results. University of Kentucky researchers examined the results of four studies on meal-replacement bars and shakes involving 470 women and 133 men. The participants were encouraged to use meal-replacement products twice a day for six months.

At the end of the study, the average female participant lost 9.3 percent of her initial body weight, or about 17 pounds. The average male participant lost 8.6 percent, or about 19 pounds.

The research also found that meal replacements demand less intervention than other weight-loss plans. That means fewer hours of weight-loss instruction and fewer visits to the doctor or diet counselor.

Researchers concluded that meal replacements are effective weight-loss tools. Just remember — your success depends on the number of calories you consume and your faithfulness to the diet plan.

Do your homework before buying. One dilemma dieters face is the huge variety of available products. A grocery store's nutrition section can be bewildering. There are shakes and bars for energy, protein, diet, and meal replacement.

To make matters worse, you have to choose among "energy-restricted," "low-carb," and "very low-carb" products. The differences aren't always clear.

Do some research before you shop so you'll know what to look for. You could also ask your doctor or nutritionist for advice. In addition, don't overlook some of these products' common shortcomings.

▶ Their nutrition labels are known to be suspect, sometimes underreporting carbohydrates, saturated fat, and sodium.

▶ They're very low in dietary fiber, which is important for good health.

▶ They may contain ingredients you don't want, like herbs or stimulants such as caffeine.

Be sensible and keep this in mind – the best way to lose weight is to burn more calories than you take in by practicing portion control and getting regular physical activity.

When to consider weight-loss surgery

Weight-loss surgery isn't the answer for people who want an easy way to lose 10 or 20 pounds. Only people who are 100 pounds or more overweight or people 85 to 100 pounds overweight who have obesity-related medical problems, including type 2 diabetes, should consider this surgery – and only if other weight-loss treatments have failed.

Weight reduction, or bariatric, surgery increased from 36,700 cases in 2000 to 171,000 in 2005. A rise in the number of obese people, improved surgical techniques, and a number of high-profile success stories are responsible for the rise. It seems to work – most people lose about two-thirds of their excess weight within two years, and most enjoy better health. Here are two types of weight-loss surgery.

Laparoscopic gastric banding. In this procedure, an adjustable silicone band is placed around the upper part of your stomach. This makes your stomach smaller so you can't eat as much, and you feel full faster. This procedure has several benefits, like less time in surgery, a shorter hospital stay, and fewer complications after surgery. The band can also be removed. On the downside, there is very little information about its long-term effectiveness. Gastric banding costs about $18,000.

Gastric bypass. With bypass surgery, a pouch about the size of an egg is created in your upper stomach, and the small intestine is attached to it. You feel full faster, and food bypasses most of the stomach and upper intestine. That means fewer calories are absorbed, which leads to weight loss. This operation costs about $25,000 to $30,000 – if there are no complications. Although this surgery has a better record for both losing weight and keeping it off,

Shrink your stomach naturally

Desperate dieters demand extreme measures. Some people find controlling their appetites so difficult they have their stomachs surgically stapled so they'll eat less and lose weight. But there's no need to have surgery to shed pounds. Your stomach will shrink naturally — if you just put less food into it.

The trick is to stick to a regular meal plan — typically one that focuses on eating smaller meals more frequently. Remember, just because you eat more meals doesn't mean you should get more calories. You simply divide those calories more evenly throughout the day so you're less likely to get hungry and overeat. You want to avoid large meals and stuffing yourself because you'll undo all your good work and increase your stomach size again.

it's a more difficult procedure with a higher risk of complications, like nutritional deficiencies.

Medicare has recently eased its criteria for paying for these surgeries and other insurers are expected to follow suit. Check your health insurance plan to see if it covers weight-loss surgery.

Follow your nose to a slimmer you

Throw those deprivation diets out the door. Dr. Alan Hirsch says he's discovered the secret to slimming down and staying that way. His formula for success? Your nose.

You stop eating when the satiety center in your brain is satisfied. And you satisfy the satiety center in your brain in a big way through your sense of smell, according to Hirsch, the Neurological Director of the Smell and Taste Research Foundation in Chicago and author of *Dr. Hirsch's Guide To Scentsational Weight Loss.*

If your nose and satiety center are working well together, your brain can determine the amount of food you've eaten by the amount of odors that reached your satiety center via your nose. However, Hirsch and his team of researchers have also found that it's possible to fool your satiety center just by smelling certain scents. The scents they've found to be most helpful are peppermint, green apple, and banana. Some herb shops and drugstores carry these scents.

People who participated in trials to test the scent theory lost an average of 5 pounds a month without restricting food or engaging in a lot of exercise. The scents simply helped their satiety center register fullness faster so they ate less and lost weight.

Smelling the scents before you eat and anytime you have a craving can dramatically reduce your calorie consumption. Each time you use the scents, sniff three times in each nostril. Switch odors every day. If you become bored with the smells, they're less likely to be effective.

Even though you're eating less, don't deprive yourself of food. Eat three small meals and two small snacks every day. Otherwise, you'll likely get so hungry you'll end up stuffing yourself, which defeats the purpose of using the scents.

The only side effect so far from this smell therapy has been excess weight loss. However, the researchers do caution that people with asthma or people who have migraines triggered by different odors probably shouldn't participate in this particular weight-loss plan.

Outsmart sugar cravings with super snacks

Sugar cravings can derail even the most carefully planned diet. In particular, if you have diabetes you know you can't ignore between-meal hunger pains. But if you substitute these healthy munchies for sweet heavy-hitters, you can snack yourself thin.

▶ Eat an apple or a handful of baby carrots between meals. Naturally sweet, they can tide you over to the next meal.

▶ Add protein, like cottage cheese or peanut butter, to your snack to feel full longer.

▶ Reach for peanuts. Unlike most salty foods, peanuts will not make you crave sugar. They're protein-rich and satisfying.

▶ Air-pop your own popcorn and flavor it with spices. This is a fiber-rich, low-cal alternative to sweets.

▶ Measure out a handful of unsalted pretzels. They're lower in fat than many other snacks.

▶ Stay away from the cookie jar. Keep some crunchy vegetables, like celery, cut up in your fridge.

▶ Chew sugar-free gum. A recent study found that chewing gum increases the number of calories you burn by 20 percent.

▶ Substitute beverages like black or green tea for sugary sodas. According to one belief, switching to tea as your only beverage may help you drop pounds. The caffeine is thought to speed up your metabolism, helping you burn fat faster.

Dodge disease the Asian way

The humble life of a peasant may not be for you, but eating like one could save your heart and your health. In the China-Cornell-Oxford Diet and Health Project, the largest study of its kind, researchers charted the eating habits of more than 10,000 Chinese people, who happen to have amazingly low cholesterol levels and heart disease risk. Asians from other countries also enjoy uncommon protection from illnesses as diverse as cancer, heart disease, diabetes, and obesity.

Opt for orange juice

Research suggests orange juice is an effective appetite suppressant. In a Yale University study, overweight men who drank OJ before their meal ate nearly 300 fewer calories at lunch. Overweight women consumed an average of 431 fewer midday calories. Their intakes were contrasted with similarly overweight men and women who drank plain water before lunch.

To reap these benefits, drink a glass of OJ a half-hour to an hour before a meal. You'll eat fewer calories during the meal and still feel comfortably full. Just don't forget to include that glass of orange juice when figuring total calories for the day. Keep an eye on your blood sugar after you drink OJ.

Experts are now piecing together a picture of the ideal Asian diet, one full of high-fiber, nutrient-rich plant foods and low in animal products and total fat — the kind that simple, rural Asian peasants eat.

Apparently, this diet works. Even the average high cholesterol in parts of Asia is about the same as the lowest range in the United States. Heart disease accounts for only about 15 percent of deaths there, a far cry from the more than 40 percent it claims in the United States. Take the road to better health by filling your plate with these modest but magnificent foods.

Get on board with grains. Rice, wheat, millet, corn, and barley form the basis of most Asian diets. They are, however, less refined than the kind most Westerners eat, so they retain more natural fiber and other nutrients. Shop for unrefined rice to get a taste of good Asian health, and take a chance on exotic varieties, like jasmine, basmati, or brown rice.

Add in the value of vegetables. Exotic-sounding greens like bok choy, amaranth, bamboo shoots, and water spinach are second only to grains as key players in Asian diets. If you can't find these in your local store and don't have access to special markets, substitute more familiar but equally healthy vegetables like broccoli, peppers, spinach, celery, or carrots. Spice them up for added flavor and a true taste of the Orient.

Make way for fruits. Fresh fruits appear frequently at Asian meals. In fact, they're often served in place of desserts and sweets, a far better choice than the high-sugar, high-fat treats Westerners often indulge in. Stay away from sugary sweets for a while and see if your taste buds take a liking to naturally sweet fruits.

Don't forget legumes. Asians understand the importance of the basic bean. They make soybeans into tofu, paste, noodles, sheets, and they even eat them plain. Because people in this part of the world eat few animal foods, beans fill their protein requirements. In addition, legumes are loaded with fiber, phytoestrogens, and other nutrients. Whether you dip into unusual legumes, like chickpeas, lentils, and mung beans, or stick to old standbys, be sure you make them a regular part of your meals for an authentic Asian diet.

Nibble on nuts and seeds. Pine nuts, almonds, walnuts, and cashews are just a few nuts you'll see gracing Asian dishes. Whether chopped and sprinkled over food, or crushed in sauces and dressings, eating a handful of nuts and seeds every day goes a long way toward total health. They are generally loaded with unsaturated fat, vitamin E, and ellagic acid, and they help lower cholesterol, fight cancer, and boost your brainpower.

Fill your basket with fish. These creatures of the sea are rich in omega-3 fatty acids and protein, plus they have the added boon of being low in cholesterol. They're a healthier alternative to red meat and may be one reason people in Asia have low cholesterol levels. Try fish chunked up and cooked in stir-fries and soups.

Decide for yourself about dairy. Daily milk, cheese, and yogurt simply aren't options for many people in Asia. Despite that fact, they enjoy unusually low rates of osteoporosis compared to Western countries, where calcium-rich dairy foods are eaten much more often. Some experts think a plant-based diet could contribute to their amazing bone health.

Eat less red meat, poultry, and eggs. The Asian diet includes less meat and, therefore, less animal protein than Western diets. Instead, Asian people get most of their protein from plants like legumes, nuts, and seeds. This may mean a healthier heart and arteries in the long run. To eat the Asian way, try cutting back on red meat to one serving a month, and poultry and eggs to once a week.

Weigh pros and cons of natural sweetener

Sugar is the sweetener of choice for many people. Unfortunately, it's full of empty calories. That's why stevia — which is calorie-free, tastes much sweeter than sugar, and won't raise your blood sugar — appeals to people who want to have their cake, or soft drink, and eat it, too. Too bad sweetening your food with stevia is controversial.

Look before you leap. Stevia is an extract that comes from the leaves of a South American shrub. You can use this natural sugar substitute instead of chemical artificial sweeteners, like saccharin and aspartame. Non-nutritive sweeteners make your food and drink taste good, but they don't add the calories found in sugar and high fructose corn syrup.

While it sounds great, stevia has one big drawback. The U.S. Food and Drug Administration (FDA) has not approved it. That means food manufacturers can't put it in drinks, cakes, cookies, candy, or other processed foods.

Although stevia has been widely used in Japan, Korea, and Brazil, the FDA says it doesn't have enough proof to declare it safe. It's also not allowed in Canada and parts of Europe.

Common weight-loss blunder

People with diabetes who have a sweet tooth can find ways to work sugar into their diet. But if you're trying to lose weight, you may want to substitute low-calorie sweeteners, like aspartame (Equal), saccharin (Sweet'N Low), or sucralose (Splenda). The ADA says they are safe for people with diabetes, and they don't have calories or carbohydrates. Try them to sweeten your coffee or tea.

But just because a food is sweetened with a sugar substitute doesn't mean it's a good choice for weight loss. Some processed foods, like sugar-free cookies or cheesecake, may still contain lots of calories from fat. Check the label's nutrition information so you'll know exactly what you're eating.

Check out what experts say. Research on stevia is mixed. Some studies conducted outside the United States say it's fine to use. Other studies suggest there are serious health hazards, like reproductive problems and cancer, especially if it's widely used.

University of Arizona professor emeritus Ryan Huxtable is a toxicologist whose research on stevia is highly regarded by other scientists looking for answers. Huxtable says we don't know enough about it to make a good judgment.

"Its use in other countries is beside the point," he says. "If toxicological associations are not looked for, they will not be found, even if they occur. Consider the use of tobacco for several hundred years by millions of people, without an awareness of associated health problems."

Today, smoking's relationship to cancer and other diseases is obvious, thanks to appropriate research, the professor says.

Laboratory studies show stevia could interfere with the way food is converted to energy. That's reason enough to find out what the risk is to humans, Huxtable says. He's also concerned because Americans like sweets a lot more than people in other countries. The amount of stevia used per person in the United States would likely be much more than in Asia or South America.

"Toxicity is a function of dose," he explains. Whether the side effects are worth the benefit from a substance depends on how much of it you use.

Some dangerous reactions might not show up in small-scale studies. A serious public health risk can occur when a product goes on the market and is used by millions of people without careful testing. For example, the arthritis medication Vioxx (rofecoxib) was on the market for five years before a serious association with heart disease was discovered, Huxtable says.

Make a wise choice. Just because something is "natural" doesn't mean it's safe. Until the FDA determines that stevia poses no danger, you won't find it in processed foods as a food additive. However, you can buy it at health food stores and some grocery stores as a dietary supplement. The FDA does not regulate supplements.

Slim down with a 'cheap' snack

Healthy snacks actually cost less than unhealthy ones. Researchers at the National Cancer Institute priced a serving of potato chips at about 25 cents and a serving of packaged chocolate chip cookies at 24 cents. In contrast, an apple costs about 13 cents.

Stevia is available as a liquid and a powder. You can buy it in small packets and large cans. Because it's heat resistant, it can be used for baking and cooking, just like regular sugar.

Watchdog groups like the Center for Science in the Public Interest and a United Nations expert panel have concluded that a drop or two in your tea or a little sprinkled on your cereal probably won't be enough to hurt you. But they don't endorse wide use of this controversial sweetener. If you have diabetes, talk to your doctor before you use it.

5 reasons to avoid 100-calorie snack packs

You've probably noticed the rise in snack foods packaged in 100-calorie servings. Cookies, chips, pretzels — many of your favorite goodies are available in small servings that limit the number of calories in a splurge. These small packs may be great for helping control how much you eat, but they aren't a cure-all for a bad diet. Consider these drawbacks.

▶ Small serving size. You may not feel you've had enough. If you're used to traditional single-serving portions of chips or cookies, you'll be sadly disappointed by these packs, many of which contain just 18 to 24 grams of food.

▶ High price. Sometimes eating goodies from 100-calorie packs means you pay more than twice the price for the same product. Try making your own snack packs by purchasing a large box of the same item, then dividing them into small baggies.

▶ Hidden fat. Even if these processed foods say they contain 0 grams of trans fats in a serving, they actually may have up to 0.49 grams. These half-grams add up if you turn to the same snacks repeatedly.

▶ Few nutrients. Think about what you are missing. You can get more food and loads of vitamins and minerals for the same 100 calories if you choose a medium banana, 1 1/2 ounces of light string cheese, or a small serving of low-fat yogurt.

▶ Unhealthy choices. Small is not the same as healthy. If you buy regular potato chips in 100-calorie packs, you're still eating potato chips – just fewer of them. A better option may be to buy baked chips or those with less fat, then make your own small packs.

Serve tasty feasts minus high-calorie fat

You've heard all about how dietary fat is high in calories – 1 gram of fat has 9 calories. On top of that, certain fats can harm your body, especially your heart. Now it's time to take action. Trimming fat from your diet is a good place to start, but it's not enough. You also need to replace the unhealthy saturated and trans fats with the heart-loving family of mono- and polyunsaturated fats.

You'll find saturated fats in meat, egg yolks, cream, whole milk, butter, and cheese, as well as a few vegetable fats like coconut oil, palm oil, and hydrogenated vegetable shortenings. Trans fats are often lurking in processed foods, like cookies and crackers.

Safflower oil, sunflower oil, and soybean oil are high in polyunsaturated fats, while olive oil and canola oil are high in monounsaturated fats.

Begin making the switch to replace the harmful fats with healthy ones. Aim for these leaner, meaner meats and meat replacements.

▶ Favor fish and poultry over red and processed meats.

▶ Eat beans, peas, lentils, and nuts instead of meat.

▶ Choose turkey over other types of luncheon meat since it's usually lower in fat.

▶ Limit the amount of liver, kidneys, and other organ meats you eat.

Add zing with lemon juice

Sun-drenched lemon juice adds fat-free flavor with a healthy dose of vitamin C. You can even buy it in a portable squeeze bottle so you can take it everywhere you go. Switch from fatty sauces to lemon juice when you season vegetables, fish, or lean meat. Make a lively, reduced-fat dressing with vinegar, a bit of olive oil, a splash of lemon juice, and some Italian herbs. Replace butter with lemon juice to rev up the flavor of vegetables. Or top baked potatoes with a whipped mixture of lemon juice and low-fat cottage cheese.

▶ Buy the leanest cuts of meat you can afford. Select beef cuts with the word loin or round, and pork with the word loin or leg in the name. Go with choice instead of prime meats, and choose those labeled USDA Select.

▶ Pick low-fat versions if you must eat processed meats, like sausage, bacon, and bologna.

▶ Substitute small amounts of olive oil for butter or margarine. If you use margarine, buy one made with liquid vegetable oil.

▶ Use part-skim mozzarella cheese instead of high-fat cheeses, like cheddar or Swiss.

3 unusual causes of weight gain

Eating too much food is not always the reason behind your weight gain. Though relatively rare, there are three other causes you might want to ask your doctor about.

▶ Thyroid problems. Your thyroid controls how fast you use energy. If it produces too little thyroid hormone, a condition called hypothyroidism, you can gain weight. Ask your doctor for a simple blood test if you regularly feel cold and fatigued.

▶ Heredity. Genetics can play a strong role in weight gain. You could have too little of the hormone that signals you are full. You may also have a metabolism that processes fat too efficiently, which means you store it away like a squirrel before winter.

▶ Medications. Weight gain can be a side effect of some antidepressants and estrogen, as well as drugs used to treat blood

pressure and diabetes — among many other conditions. Don't stop taking your medication. Share your concerns about your weight with your doctor. She may recommend a similar drug without this side effect.

Read between the lines for healthy snacking

"Low fat!" "Made with real fruit!" "Lite!" Food labels on every kind of snack scream about their goodness. Unfortunately, some

---

Drown a snack attack in popcorn

After-lunch sleepiness can trigger a bout of mid-afternoon munchies. But air-popped popcorn with a tiny dash of olive oil might keep you away from the vending machine and its dieting dangers. Popcorn can make you feel twice as full as a candy bar because it scores well on the satiety index — an index created by researchers to show which foods keep you feeling full longest.

---

so-called healthy food can lead to weight gain as easily as the junk it replaces in your pantry.

Take low-fat foods. You may think since they're lower in fat, they are also much lower in calories. In reality, they typically contain only 30 fewer calories per serving than their regular-fat counterparts. However, people in one study ate nearly 30 percent more when they knew they were eating a low-fat snack. Overweight people ate almost 50 percent more.

Mistakes like these can ruin your diet. These five rules can help save it.

▶ Read the nutrition labels on food. Look for snacks with the most nutrients and the fewest calories, and check both the sugar and fat content.

▶ Grab several brands of the same item when shopping, and choose the one with the fewest calories, not just the least fat.

▶ Check the serving size on the nutrition label. Sometimes manufacturers try to make a food's nutrition numbers look better — less fat or fewer calories — by basing them on ridiculously small servings.

▶ Make sure good-for-you foods, like vegetables, weren't prepared with butter, cream, or breading.

▶ Choose naturally low-fat, nutrient-rich foods, like fresh, unprocessed fruits and vegetables over processed, prepackaged "healthy" snacks.

50 nutrition tips to keep you slim and healthy

Dieting doesn't have to be an all-or-nothing endeavor. You can tackle a weight problem by making small changes in the way you eat. These little fixes add good nutrition so you can make the most of your calories.

▶ Put spinach on your sandwich instead of lettuce. A recent study found most people couldn't tell the difference, and spinach is much more nutritious.

▶ Eat your garnish. Restaurants often pretty up your plate with parsley or kale. Instead of admiring these nutritional powerhouses, eat them.

▶ Toss some blueberries in your morning cereal, muffin or pancake mix, or even in a bowl of ice cream.

▶ Try mashed avocado as a spread instead of mayonnaise, butter, or cream cheese.

▶ Use olive oil or canola oil instead of animal oils or other vegetable oils.

▶ Invest in a good set of nonstick cookware. You'll be able to use less fat when cooking.

▶ Use legumes (beans and peas) in soups and casseroles, and cut back on meat.

▶ Choose lean cuts of meat, and trim away as much excess fat as you can before cooking.

▶ Don't smother your baked potato with butter or sour cream. Instead, try topping it with salsa or low-fat chili.

▶ Sauté vegetables in wine or broth instead of butter or oil.

▶ Add mashed avocado or pumpkin to mashed potatoes for a little extra nutrition. Use about one-fourth to one-half cup for every two cups of potatoes.

▶ Serve sweet foods warm. Heat enhances the sweet taste of foods, so you may be able to add less sugar.

▶ Make yogurt "cheese." It's a good substitute for sour cream. Line a strainer or funnel with cheesecloth or a paper coffee filter. Add plain yogurt and let it drain into a bowl overnight in the refrigerator. Simply discard the liquid, and you're ready to use the yogurt in your favorite recipe.

Maintenance strategies that really work

Maintaining your weight is just as important as losing weight — and often as difficult. But it doesn't have to be. When it comes to taking it off and keeping it off, focus on weight-loss strategies that work for a lifetime. According to data from the National Weight Control Registry, people who have succeeded at losing and maintaining weight limit fast foods to less than once a week, weigh themselves regularly, eat five times a day, and burn an average of 400 calories a day through exercise.

When losing weight, you must burn more calories than you take in. It's important to keep an eye on your calories even after you reach your desired weight. Work off the same number of calories you take in, and your weight will stay the same.

▶ Chill soups and stews so most of the fat will solidify on top. Skim off the solid fat, and then heat and eat the lighter soup.

▶ Choose fruits and vegetables with the darkest colors to get the most vitamin C.

▶ Order your pizza with lots of veggies, and blot with a paper towel to absorb any excess grease.

▶ Add shredded apple to a peanut butter or grilled cheese sandwich.

▶ Throw vegetables on the grill at your next cookout. Skewer chunks of onion, green pepper, tomatoes, and mushrooms, or cook up some asparagus spears.

▶ Grill a tropical kabob with chunks of pineapple, papaya, and ham.

▶ Bake a banana. Put a whole, ripe banana on a cookie sheet. Bake for 20 minutes at 350 degrees. Split the skin and sprinkle with nutmeg or cinnamon.

▶ Stuff bell peppers with cooked rice or pasta and tomato sauce. Cook in a muffin tin to help the peppers hold their shape.

▶ Mix chopped kiwi or papaya with tomatoes, green onions, and cilantro for salsa with a surprising sweet twist.

▶ Purée mangoes and use as a sauce for grilled chicken, pork, or fish.

▶ Make a yummy and attractive breakfast parfait. Layer low-fat yogurt, granola cereal, and fruit such as peaches or pineapple in a parfait glass.

Clever way to feel full longer

Psyllium, the husk of the plantago plant's seed, may work well as an appetite suppressant. In a small study of 17 women, those who took 20 grams of plantago seed granules along with a glass of water three hours before a meal felt significantly fuller one hour after the meal than women who had taken a placebo (fake psyllium). In addition, the women who used the psyllium ate less fat.

Researchers think psyllium works as an appetite suppressant because it holds water and swells, creating a feeling of fullness. Although the evidence supporting psyllium as a weight-loss aid is scant, you may want to try it. Consuming psyllium won't harm you unless you take more than recommended or are allergic to it. Other benefits include regularity and cholesterol control. You can find psyllium seeds at most health food stores.

▶ Buy canned fruit packed in its own juice — not in calorie-laden syrup.

▶ Don't skip breakfast. If you're in a hurry, grab an apple, a bagel, or a banana.

▶ Bake your own bread and add dried fruits, vegetables, or seeds for more taste and nutrition.

▶ Look for 100-percent fruit juice. Other fruit drinks usually contain more sugar than nutrition.

▶ Eat broth-based soups. They are far lower in fat than cream-based alternatives.

▶ Serve meat or poultry with cranberry sauce, salsa, or chutney, and skip the gravy.

▶ Don't let dining out become an excuse for pigging out. Most restaurants serve unnecessarily large portions. Split an entrée with someone else, or eat only half and ask for a doggie bag.

▶ Read labels carefully. Don't be fooled by fat-free foods. Many of them are still high in calories.

▶ Try angel food cake topped with fresh fruit when you just have to eat cake.

▶ Hold the butter. Popcorn can be a high-fiber, low-calorie snack if you don't drench it in butter. If you don't like air-popped corn, try using a small amount of olive oil for a delicious healthy flavor.

▶ Go easy on nuts. They tend to be high in fat, but they also get high marks for nutrition. Include them in your diet — just don't overdo it.

▶ Focus on your food. You'll eat less and enjoy your food more if you don't eat while working, watching television, or driving.

▶ Add brown or wild rice to casseroles and soups for more fiber and nutrition.

▶ Substitute mung bean paste for some of the butter in peanut butter cookies to lower fat and increase fiber.

▶ Try exotic fruit, like kiwis or mangoes, if you are bored with bananas but want the potassium.

▶ Microwave your vegetables to retain more of their vitamins and minerals.

▶ Toss steamed veggies with whole-wheat pasta to add more fiber to your diet.

▶ Grill fish by wrapping in foil with a little lemon juice and herbs.

▶ Blend up a fast, nutritious shake with low-fat milk, low-fat yogurt, ice cubes, and your favorite fruit.

▶ Bypass self-basting turkeys, which are injected with fat to make them moist. Baste your turkey with broth instead.

▶ Substitute unsweetened applesauce for up to half the butter or oil called for in your baking recipes.

▶ Sprinkle flaxseed on soups, salads, and hot or cold cereals.

▶ Ask for sauces and salad dressings on the side when dining out, and then use them sparingly.

▶ Broil, bake, grill, steam, or poach meats and vegetables instead of frying or boiling them. You'll lower fat and retain nutrients.

▶ Replace the cream in your recipe with low-fat sour cream or low-fat evaporated milk.

▶ Choose sun-dried tomatoes over the fresh variety for more lycopene. Those packed in oil are best at helping your body absorb this cancer-fighting nutrient.

The Stress Connection

Curb anxiety to lower blood sugar

Balance blood sugar with biofeedback

Everyone experiences rough times in life, but some people don't handle stress well. If you're dealing with the grief of losing a loved one or the uncertainty of moving to a new area, brace yourself for the possibility of another life-changing event – diabetes.

A Dutch study of more than 2,000 middle-age people found a relationship between major stressful events within the past five years and an increased risk of diabetes.

Simple way to find peace of mind

You know the feeling you get when you're dreading something. Your heart starts pounding, and your hands get sweaty. Those feelings of anxiety are natural reactions to stressful situations.

When you're in trouble, your body releases adrenaline and cortisol, hormones that prepare you to deal with emergencies. Once your adrenaline is pumping, your body heats up to generate all the energy and strength you'll need for a crisis. When the threat is gone, your body rests and recovers.

Problems arise when everyday stressors keep you in this mode all the time. You may even suffer from an anxiety disorder that causes constant, unexplainable feelings of dread. If your body never gets a chance to rest, wear-and-tear sets in. Chronic anxiety can weaken your mind, bones, heart, and immune system.

Beat stress by giving yourself time to enjoy doing what you love. Whether it's gardening or bird watching, your hobby helps you relax, which can help prevent future illness.

Researchers say experiencing things like the death of a spouse, serious financial trouble, or the end of a relationship may tamper with your body's ability to regulate certain hormones. The people in the study with the highest number of stressful events were 60 percent more likely to develop diabetes than those with fewer events. If you're facing traumatic incidents, seek professional help for ways to handle the stress.

Here's a simple way to regulate your blood sugar, heart rate, blood pressure, circulation, and digestion – and perhaps your stress levels, too. Biofeedback teaches you how to recognize and control changes in your body. It has helped treat conditions ranging from constipation to heart rhythm abnormalities to depression. Biofeedback may also give you power over your physical reaction to stress.

Researchers tested people with type 2 diabetes to see how biofeedback and relaxation therapy could help control high blood sugar. People who tried these relaxation methods for three months had better blood sugar control and less muscle tension than those in a control group. In fact, those in the biofeedback group enjoyed nearly a 10-percent drop in blood sugar.

Any gadget that provides information about your body can be a biofeedback device. For example, if you try relaxation therapy to lower blood pressure and ease stress, a blood pressure cuff can show you when it is working. More advanced biofeedback devices may monitor brain waves or measure muscle tension.

You'll need a trained biofeedback specialist and the right equipment to learn to control physical properties like brain waves. But you can teach yourself to monitor your breathing and heart rate – and concentrate on returning them to normal when stress strikes.

9 easy ways to improve your quality of life

You know stress wreaks havoc on your health – in fact, it impacts almost every system in your body. That's why, if you have diabetes, you must go beyond managing your diet, weight, and blood sugar, and take care of your mental health, too.

Finding ways to cope with daily stress is essential to learning how to feel better now. It will help you be there for your loved ones tomorrow, and free your mind from worry. It's not about being hungry or knocking yourself out. It's about enjoying your life.

Here are some cutting-edge theories from top scientists to help you de-stress.

Let faith bring you peace. There is a growing amount of scientific research that shows people with a strong, active religious life are healthier, often live longer, and generally deal better with life's difficulties than those who are nonreligious. Many find believing in a higher power to be an immense source of comfort and peace. These people are usually more optimistic about the future because they believe events are part of a bigger plan. Having what is called a

Snack on strawberries for serenity

You don't have to take tranquilizers to feel calmer. Strawberries can reduce stress and calm anxiety by giving you a surge of dopamine, an ingredient in the natural brain chemical norepinephrine. This chemical controls how well you deal with stress. Although the link has only been shown in animals, it can't hurt to eat a few strawberries when you're feeling anxious.

"prayerful, prayerlike" attitude – one of devotion and acceptance – can help you deal with stress.

Stay close to family and friends. Loved ones touch your heart in many ways. Amazing research about relationships and longevity shows a large support group lowers stress levels, blood pressure, and your risk of heart disease and heart attacks. Face it, having friends and family around can mean a healthier, longer life. If you're happily married, odds are you'll live longer and have fewer medical problems than your single, widowed, or divorced counterparts. Not only are spouses a great source of support and social fun, they tend to watch out for your health, ensuring that both of you get the best medical care. Men, especially, seem to benefit from being married.

Loosen tense muscles. Just like ice cream heads straight for the hips, stress tends to get trapped in tight muscles. For example, holding on to stress can cause crippling back and shoulder pain. To release your muscles, try simple progressive relaxation.

▶ Find a comfortable position and begin breathing slowly and deeply.

▶ Tense the muscles in your toes for a count of 10.

▶ Release them slowly and completely while you count to 10.

▶ Next, tense the muscles of your feet in the same way.

▶ Continue up the entire length of your body, tensing and relaxing every muscle group.

▶ By the time you reach the top of your head, you should feel completely relaxed.

Let laughter into your life. The cheapest medicine around – a bout of good humor – can put pain and problems in perspective. Studies show laughter lowers stress levels and boosts your immune system.

▶ Laughter can relieve pain, but humor works best if you choose your own "medicine." So pick out your favorite comedy the next time you visit the video store and laugh your pain away.

▶ Joke fall flat? Laugh anyway. Even forced laughter will improve your mood.

▶ Check the TV listings for good comedies a week in advance. Anticipating mirth boosts your immune system about as much as the actual laughing does.

Reach out to others. Variety may not only be the spice of life, it seems to mean a longer life, too. Take this advice to heart and widen your circle to include those outside your normal social group. Nurture friendships with teens and young adults. Their youth and enthusiasm will keep you young, just as your wisdom can help them grow. Consider volunteering or mentoring if you find yourself isolated from new people. Whether it's church or a weekly card game, being involved in a community keeps you connected and optimistic. Socializing this way is also associated with fewer deaths from all causes combined.

Be mindful of the moment. When was the last time you noticed the tickle of peach fuzz on your lips, or how socks feel on your feet? Stress crops up when you worry about the future. If you can focus on the moment, the future and its problems will melt away. A practical example of this is called mindfulness, which requires you notice and accept the sensations and thoughts you experience as they happen.

This can be easier than you think. Start by learning how to really pay attention to your breathing.

▶ Relax and follow your breath in and out. Notice the beginning, middle, and end of each in-breath.

▶ Do the same with each out-breath. Notice the rise and fall of your chest or abdomen. Don't try to breathe any differently from your normal breathing.

▶ Continue breathing slowly and evenly – with awareness – for 10 to 20 minutes.

Now practice this same mindfulness during your everyday activities. Chew your food slowly, for example, tasting every bite, and notice the different textures in your mouth. Experts believe mindfulness can

Quick tips for beating the blahs

Some forms of serious depression require drug treatment from your doctor. With a milder case of the blues, simple changes in behavior or activities may be enough to lift that cloud.

▶ Get regular exercise.

▶ Listen to music.

▶ Stop smoking.

▶ Get enough protein and iron in your diet.

▶ Ask your doctor if a nutritional supplement called SAMe is right for you.

▶ Eat fish, flaxseed, or walnuts for omega-3 fatty acids.

▶ Spend time with friends and family.

▶ Get enough deep, restful sleep.

▶ Set short-term goals.

▶ Seek treatment for any health issues.

▶ Get some sunshine every day.

▶ Give to others by volunteering.

bring on positive changes in how your brain and immune system respond to stress and disease.

Opt for optimism. If you're an optimist, you know you have whatever it takes to make it through tough times. You don't paste on a happy face and ignore sorrow or trouble. In fact, you probably feel deeply. You simply control the intensity of those feelings – not allowing them to overwhelm you. Perhaps because of this positive attitude, optimists tend to live longer than pessimists. If looking for that silver lining doesn't come naturally, don't be discouraged. You can learn to be an optimist. Here are a few tricks to get you started.

▶ Smile. If you turn on a high-wattage grin – one that raises your cheeks – you'll really feel happier. Research proves your emotions follow your expression, not the other way around.

▶ Resist negative thoughts. See yourself as a success, and failure will become the exception rather than the rule.

▶ Put it all in perspective. Ask yourself if this will matter in five years.

▶ If you catch yourself too often thinking, "I wish I were a ...," try finishing this sentence instead, "I'm glad I'm not a ... ." By comparing yourself to others who are less fortunate, you create a more positive, satisfied view of your life.

Learn to forgive. Letting go of anger and resentment is good for your mind and your body. According to research, if you forgive:

▶ you'll suffer less stress and depression and their unhealthy symptoms.

▶ you'll have generally fewer health problems.

▶ you'll feel better psychologically and emotionally.

▶ you'll increase your self-confidence and enjoy better relationships.

Holding on to this kind of pain doesn't harm the person who wronged you, but your body's response – a rise in blood pressure, anxiety levels, and stress – may increase your risk of heart disease and cancer.

Remember, forgiveness doesn't necessarily mean you reconcile with the person who hurt you, or that you do not pursue justice. It means you let go of the blame and the pain. This way you regain power over your own emotions.

Make a furry friend. A dog is man's best friend for a reason. The unconditional love from a pet, and the physical touch you lavish on it can both reduce stress. But you don't have to stick with just dogs. Even a goldfish can calm you down and improve your mood.

Smart ways to fall asleep faster

Worrying about problems and planning for the next day can keep you awake at night. Researchers tested various behavioral methods, or ways of changing how you think about sleep, and pitted them against taking sleeping pills. They looked at progressive muscle relaxation, biofeedback, cognitive behavioral therapy (CBT), and other techniques.

Taking drugs to bring on sleep works. Unfortunately, it's not as fast as behavioral changes, and people can come to rely on sleeping pills. Scientists say changing people's thoughts can actually cure insomnia in the long run, unlike drugs. In one study, researchers found CBT – talk therapy with a counselor – worked better than sleeping pills for people with chronic insomnia.

You can seek help from a professional, or you can try to improve your own thought patterns. Pay attention to your beliefs about sleep and sleeplessness. Try to change negative thoughts like, "I'll never survive tomorrow if I don't get to sleep soon," to positive ideas like, "I'll bet I'm actually getting more rest than I think." Don't get preoccupied by the idea of insomnia, and don't watch the minutes tick by as you lie awake.

Finally, if your thoughts are still racing ahead to tomorrow's problems, get up and write down the trouble that's keeping you awake. Sometimes putting it on paper can put your mind at rest.

Warning signs of nerve damage

Neuropathy, or nerve damage from high blood sugar, comes in three different forms.

Sensory, or peripheral, neuropathy is damage to nerves that carry feeling from your body to your brain. At first, you're likely to feel pain and numbness or tingling in your hands and feet. Eventually, you're unable to feel heat, cold, or even pain in those body parts.

Autonomic neuropathy affects nerves that control the involuntary functions of your body — particularly relating to your heart, lungs, stomach, intestines, bladder, and sex organs. It may become difficult for you to empty your bladder or digest your food. Men could become impotent.

Motor neuropathy, rare in people who have diabetes, damages nerves that send messages to your muscles. You could have trouble walking or moving your fingers.

See your doctor if you develop any of these problems:

▸ nausea, vomiting, bloating, constipation, or diarrhea
▸ dizziness or fainting
▸ problems with your feet, including foot ulcers or having trouble lifting a foot
▸ impotence

13 secrets for sounder sleep

People diagnosed with diabetes often take the news hard, worrying about how the disease will affect how they live. Such stress is understandable, since diabetes can cause you to make great changes, from what and when you eat to starting an exercise program to checking your blood sugar and taking drugs. It's enough to keep you up at night.

But losing sleep is the last thing you should do if you have diabetes. Experts believe sleep is necessary for your body to process sugar properly. A recent study showed people who don't get enough sleep are more likely to become resistant to insulin – a direct path to diabetes. Strive for at least eight hours of snooze time. You'll wake up with a refreshed mind and body, ready for another day of taking care of your good health.

What can you do to safeguard your sleep? First, determine if you have a problem. How well do you feel during the day? Are you energetic and alert? If so, you're probably fine. If you feel tired and irritable in the daytime or need to nap frequently, you may have a sleep problem. Most people are not aware of how often or why they awaken in the night.

Look at how you feel during the day. Take note of when you go to sleep, how long before you fall asleep, and when you wake up. Look at your eating habits. What and when do you eat or drink during the day? Try to count how many times you awaken in the night. Record times you take medication.

Ask yourself if you have more trouble falling asleep, staying asleep, or waking too early. If you have trouble falling asleep, the problem might be in your lifestyle habits like eating or drinking. It could also be from stress, worry, or shift changes.

If you have trouble staying asleep, look at underlying medical conditions, sleep apnea, restless legs syndrome, or psychological problems like depression. Then see if some of these sleep tips help solve your problem.

Set a regular schedule. You sleep according to an internal body clock known as circadian rhythms. Even the smallest changes in light, body temperature, mealtimes, and daytime activities can throw your internal sleep/wake clock out of whack.

Exercise in the afternoon. One study found 45 minutes of aerobic exercise three times a week increased deep sleep and human growth hormone (HGH). Afternoon exercise raises body temperature in the daytime, which can increase deep sleep at night. Take care not to exercise too close to bedtime. That will keep you awake.

Take a hot bath. One study found women older than 60 who took a hot bath (105 degrees F) one hour before bedtime increased deep sleep.

Watch your naps. Avoid oversleeping in the morning and don't take late afternoon or evening naps. If you have to nap, the best hours are between noon and 2 p.m. You can still get some deep sleep time during those hours.

Ditch the tobacco. If you smoke, don't do it for three to five hours before bed. Nicotine acts as a stimulant. This not only robs you of restorative sleep, but also stimulates REM sleep, which may be why you have those bizarre dreams.

Improve your sleep environment. Keep your bedroom quiet, dark, and cool. Also, your bedroom should only be used for sleeping and sex.

Try adjusting the light. Researchers have found that even normal levels of indoor artificial lighting can affect your internal clock. So in the evening, dim the lights before winding down.

Get out of bed if you're not sleepy. If you're far too alert to sleep, don't lie there and agonize. Get up and do something for a while before attempting to sleep again.

Try relaxation. Did you wake up this morning feeling like you had been run over by a train? Had you been up half the night worrying? Maybe deep sleep's magic fingers didn't have time to perform any healing miracles. Studies show stress is a deep-sleep spoiler. It's a vicious cycle. Stress disrupts your sleep, which makes you feel sleepy and irritable. This ruins your daytime performance, which leads to more stress. This ruins your sleep, and on it goes. So try relaxation techniques, such as meditation, to get your mind off your worries before bed.

Watch what you eat. Avoid spicy or heavy foods and large quantities of liquids in the evening. You might find yourself waking to urinate frequently, or you may wake to discomforts of stomach acid.

Make sure you're getting enough air. Heavy snoring; nighttime gasping, choking, or snorting; excess upper body weight; and daytime fatigue and sleepiness provide clues to sleep apnea. Sleep laboratories or sleep monitoring equipment can help determine if you have a problem. You may just need an oral appliance that helps keep your airways open during sleep.

Lose extra weight. If snoring or sleep apnea is your problem, you may need to lose some extra weight. One study found losing weight – even as little as 10 pounds – can cure snoring completely.

Limit alcohol and caffeine. Caffeine is a stimulant, so avoid drinking caffeine-containing coffee or soft drinks after noon. Don't drink alcohol three to five hours before bedtime. Not only does alcohol disrupt your sleep, it plays havoc on REM sleep. Alcohol – especially in the evening – is also a bad idea for people with diabetes.

Unwind with chamomile tea

Drink a cup of chamomile tea to relieve stress naturally. This hot beverage is so relaxing the scent alone may help calm your nerves. It's an old favorite to help you get to sleep. You can find chamomile tea in any grocery store, or make your own by steeping the herb's dried flowering heads in boiling water. When they steep, the heads release a blue oil full of chemicals called flavonoids. These chemicals affect the same receptors in your brain as prescription drugs, like Valium. You'll feel relaxed right away without suffering side effects from a drug.

Unusual ways to silence snoring

People joke about snoring, but it's not as harmless as they think. Sleep experts know it not only causes insomnia but also may be a sign of more serious health problems, including type 2 diabetes. Incredibly, researchers have found frequent snoring may double your risk for this serious condition.

Being overweight puts you at risk for both snoring and diabetes, so it makes sense they may be linked. A Swedish study of more than 2,500 men supported this connection. It found obese snorers were more likely to develop diabetes within 10 years.

But if your weight is normal, you're still not in the clear. Data from the 25-year Nurses' Health Study suggests snorers have a higher risk of diabetes no matter how much they weigh. Researchers think you get less oxygen when you snore, triggering a chain reaction that leads to insulin resistance and, eventually, diabetes.

Snoring may lead to other major health problems as well, such as sleep apnea, high blood pressure, heart disease, and stroke. You could try fixing your problem with an over-the-counter drug or device, but why not try something natural first?

Sing in the shower. About 20 minutes of singing a day could be all it takes to cure your snoring, according to a small but innovative British study. Researchers say daily singing exercises seem to tighten the throat muscles and reduce snoring. After three months, study participants who followed the recommended program snored less than before.

Sleep upright to fight gravity. In a study of astronauts and sleep problems, zero gravity appeared to help them breathe easier and enjoy a heavenly night's slumber. This leads researchers to believe gravity has a hand in snoring, especially when you lie on your back.

Try to avoid sleeping on your back, and raise yourself up by propping your back or head with pillows. You can also raise your bed by putting blocks of wood under the headboard.

Get some rest with ginger. This snore-silencing remedy comes from Central America. Steep two teaspoons of grated ginger in cinnamon tea. Then add honey and milk for flavor. Drink a cup each night before you go to bed. The theory is that ginger makes you produce more saliva, and the added moisture helps soothe your throat muscles.

Don't just roll over and close your eyes – and ears – to a snoring problem. If you and your spouse suffer through nightly "buzz saw" serenades, it's time to do something about it. Talk to your doctor about other solutions before this "harmless" problem leads to a deadly disease.

Breakfast choices: good versus bad		
	Coffee and doughnut	Oatmeal and sliced apples
What you get:	feelings of anxiety from the caffeine in your mug and almost 11 grams of fat courtesy of the doughnut	complex carbohydrates for a dose of serotonin to keep you in a good mood all day
What you miss:	your body's natural balance of blood sugar, insulin, and serotonin	coffee jitters in the morning and the 3 p.m. slump that follows

Calm your mind for a healthy body

You can't control all of your risk factors for diabetes and heart disease. For instance, you can't change your age, gender, or family history. But you can do something about the others. Is it possible to lower blood pressure, cholesterol, and blood sugar without expensive drugs? The experts say yes.

In a 12-week study at the Center for Heart Disease Prevention in Savannah, Ga., people with risk factors such as high cholesterol or high blood pressure managed to lower these levels significantly by sticking to an individually tailored exercise plan, meal plan, and other lifestyle changes.

Making these changes takes some work, but it's cheaper than drugs – without any side effects. Eating a healthy diet, exercising regularly, losing weight if you're overweight, and quitting smoking will put you on the path to a healthy heart and better control of your blood sugar – but don't stop there. Here's another important step you can take.

Learn how to handle mental stress, which can trigger a heart attack and may bring on diabetes. People with heart disease drastically lowered their risk for heart attack with four months of stress management training.

Hostility, intense arguments, and road rage have all been linked to heart attacks. Finding a healthier, more productive way to deal with stress can mean the difference between life and death. Along with stress management, try these helpful tips for better health.

▶ Laugh more. Laughter relaxes blood vessels and increases blood flow. Rent a funny movie or spend time with humorous friends or relatives.

▶ Skip the siesta. Daily afternoon naps can boost your risk of a heart attack, according to a Costa Rican study.

▶ See the glass as half full. Optimism helps ward off heart disease. A Dutch study found that optimistic men were half as likely to die from cardiovascular disease, including heart attack, stroke, and coronary heart disease, than their less optimistic counterparts.

▶ Listen to music. Italian researchers found music may have a beneficial relaxing effect on your heart.

Blast the blues with feel-good nutrients

People with diabetes have twice the risk of depression as other people. Don't ignore your moodiness, since it makes blood sugar control more difficult. But what's behind your depression? Even mild mood changes may be linked to bad eating habits. Feelings of depression are sometimes early symptoms of nutritional deficiencies, especially in older adults. This puts food on the front lines of the war on depression.

Boot the blahs with B's. B vitamins are essential to your health, but many seniors don't get enough of them. Deficiencies in vitamins B12 and B6, folate, and thiamin have all been linked to high rates of depression.

Women need to pay special attention. If you have low levels of vitamin B12, you double your risk for severe depression. In fact, a recent study found that one in four seriously depressed women were B12 deficient.

But don't despair — eat beef, turkey, chicken liver, shellfish, salmon, sardines, and trout. Just remember the National Academy of Sciences says almost one-third of seniors can't absorb the vitamin B12 in food. They suggest also eating foods fortified with this nutrient — like many commercially prepared cereals — or supplementing.

See the bright side with C. This mighty vitamin is vital in making serotonin. That means running low can leave you feeling tired and sluggish. Liven up your life by drinking a glass of orange juice or tossing slices of fresh red and green peppers in your salad.

Iron out ill humor. Just as certain vitamin deficiencies may trigger depression, so could some mineral shortages. Over 2 billion people suffer from iron-deficient anemia, a condition that can make you depressed, tired, and unable to concentrate. To ward it off, get your daily iron from dark meat, legumes, leafy green vegetables, and fortified cereals. See your doctor if you think you're anemic.

Manage moodiness with magnesium. Low moods, tiredness, confusion, and loss of appetite are symptoms of depression, but they may also be signs of a magnesium deficiency. A cup of Kellogg's bran cereal with raisins for breakfast puts you on track with more than 80 milligrams (mg) of magnesium, while a cup of cooked spinach with your dinner keeps you going with almost 160 mg. Whole grains are rich sources of this mineral, but refined grains provide little. Nuts, legumes, seafood, and dark leafy greens all pack a powerful magnesium punch.

Perk up with omega-3. Docosahexaenoic acid (DHA) and eicosapentaenoic acid (EPA) – two kinds of omega-3 fatty acids – could have lots to do with depression. Too little DHA in your body can mean too little serotonin, that important feel-good brain chemical. EPA, on the other hand, shows promise for treating some mental disorders like schizophrenia.

Fish is without question the best natural source for omega-3, followed closely by flaxseed and canola oils, wheat germ, soybeans, and nuts. Just two servings of fatty fish each week will bolster your body against depression, as well as heart attack, stroke, diabetes, and cancer.

Depression is a serious illness – you can't treat it with just diet. While eating food containing these nutrients can lower your risk of depression and speed your recovery, don't try to take on this illness alone. Look to your doctor and loved ones for help, and consider medications if your doctor recommends them.

Start now to safeguard your sex life

According to a survey conducted by the American Association of Retired Persons (AARP), 67 percent of men and 57 percent of women age 45 and older say a satisfying sexual relationship is important to their quality of life. Some health conditions, including diabetes, heart disease, or atherosclerosis (hardening of the arteries), can get in the way. In fact, about 40 percent of the men who experience impotence, or erectile dysfunction, have diabetes.

Although almost every man has a problem once in a while, impotence is defined as a consistent inability to achieve and maintain an erection sufficient for sexual intercourse. If you develop impotence, take comfort in the fact that you are not alone. About 26 out of 1,000 men ages 40 to 69 develop impotence every year.

Because your erection depends on blood flow to your penis, anything that interferes with proper blood flow can cause impotence.

Although your chances of having impotence rise as you get older, it is not an unavoidable consequence of aging.

Don't be embarrassed to talk with your doctor about sexual problems. There are many ways to treat impotence, but there are also ways to prevent it from happening in the first place. Since more than eight out of 10 cases of impotence can be traced to physical causes, taking care of yourself is one of the best ways to prevent it.

Watch the fat. High-fat foods can really foul up your sex life. Too much saturated fat and cholesterol in your diet can lead to high blood pressure and heart disease, which makes it harder for your blood vessels to get blood to where it needs to be during sex. In fact, a high total cholesterol count doubles a man's risk of becoming impotent. It's also important to know that many of the medications prescribed for high blood pressure are known to cause impotence.

Keep your weight down. Excess weight could affect your sex life beyond just having unattractive "love handles." Too much weight can contribute to diabetes and high blood pressure, two major causes of impotence.

Stop smoking. Research shows that just two cigarettes smoked before intercourse can significantly decrease blood flow to the penis. Long-term smokers are more likely to develop heart disease, which also contributes to impotence.

Limit alcohol. Drinking too much alcohol can cause even a young, healthy man to experience temporary impotence, and too much alcohol over several years can cause nerve and liver damage. This can lead to impotence that may be irreversible.

Active Living

Shape up to shake high blood sugar

2 ways to put the brakes on diabetes

You are in danger of developing type 2 diabetes and heart disease if you are in the 20 percent of Americans who have "metabolic syndrome." Metabolic syndrome is a fancy label for people with at least three of the following problems – high blood pressure, high triglyceride levels, low levels of "good" cholesterol, high blood sugar, and being overweight. You can have high blood sugar for years before you develop diabetes, a condition called prediabetes.

It's a scary trend. Experts predict the number of Americans with diabetes will triple by 2050. To avoid type 2 diabetes, follow these lifestyle changes recommended by the American Diabetes Association (ADA).

Lose some weight. If you are overweight, losing just 7 percent of your body weight, or 14 pounds for someone who weighs 200 pounds, can make a big difference. In fact, new research shows losing weight is the surest way to stop metabolic syndrome from developing into diabetes.

Get out and move. The ADA guidelines call for at least 150 minutes – two and one-half hours – of moderate exercise each week. Check with your doctor first, and pick an activity you enjoy so you'll stick with it. Research shows even people with large waistlines, who are at higher risk for type 2 diabetes, can reduce their chances of developing the disease just by becoming more active.

In fact, an 8-year study found exercise was more important in determining diabetes risk than diet, weight, or heredity. Exercise helps control your weight, which lowers your risk for diabetes, but it may also help your body process glucose. Exercise has many other important benefits as you age, such as maintaining lung capacity, retaining muscle mass and strength, and protecting your heart.

Find an activity you enjoy. It doesn't have to be strenuous. Just get moving every day. Whether you're a long-time fan of bicycling or a new convert to walking for fitness, adding activity to your day

What to do before you work out

You want to exercise wisely and safely. That's why it's a good idea to visit your doctor before starting any type of physical activity, especially if you:

▶ have diabetes or other heart disease risk factors, such as family history, smoking, or an inactive lifestyle.

▶ have a heart condition.

▶ have high blood pressure or high cholesterol, or are taking medication for either.

▶ ever experience chest pains, irregular heartbeats, or dizziness.

▶ suffer from bone or joint problems, or another chronic health problem.

Even if you're perfectly healthy, you should also check with your doctor if you're a man over age 40 or a woman over age 50 and plan to begin exercising more vigorously than usual.

can help add years to your life. The little things you do to stay active can bring lifelong health and happiness.

Slash your risk of nerve damage

Each year almost 80,000 people have a toe or foot amputated because of problems related to diabetes. In fact, aside from accidents, diabetes is the main cause of foot amputations.

About a third of all people with diabetes suffer from neuropathy, or nerve damage. Neuropathy can make your feet unable to feel heat, cold, or pain. You could step on a tack and not even feel it. High blood sugar can damage your blood vessels, causing circulation problems. If this happens, cuts, scrapes, or blisters can take a long time to heal and become infected. Eventually, the infection can spread to your bones.

Nerve damage from diabetes doesn't have to happen to you. A careful diet and exercise program can protect you.

Top tips for healthy toes

Follow these suggestions from the American Diabetes Association to keep your feet healthy.

▶ Inspect your feet daily for cuts, blisters, sores, or swelling. Get someone to help you or use a mirror if you can't see the bottoms.

▶ Have your feet checked by your doctor at least once a year — more often if you have had foot problems.

▶ Call your doctor if you have an ingrown toenail, numbness, or pain, or if you see a change in skin color.

▶ Wash and dry your feet carefully every day.

▶ Cut your toenails straight across, but file down sharp corners.

▶ Never go barefoot, even in your house.

▶ Wear shoes that fit well and don't rub.

▶ Wear socks that are soft and thick enough for extra protection.

▶ Wiggle your toes and flex your ankles while you sit to improve circulation.

Watch what you eat. The American Diabetes Association says if you can keep your blood sugar in a normal range, you'll cut in half your risk of developing neuropathy. Ask your doctor about a diet plan for losing weight and lowering blood sugar, and don't give up if you're serious about avoiding nerve damage.

Ease into exercise. The Nurses Health Study, which has followed more than 70,000 nurses for many years, says moderate exercise – such as walking an hour every day – can cut your risk of type 2 diabetes in half.

Neuropathy means taking special care of your feet during exercise. The nerves to your feet are longer than any others in your body and are more vulnerable to damage. Talk to your doctor about swimming, bicycling, rowing, or chair exercises. All these put less stress on your feet.

Check your feet before and after exercise, and be sure you don't have any blisters or cuts. Always wear shoes that fit properly – not too tight, not too loose – and comfortable, seamless socks that don't irritate your skin.

Change dangerous flab to tight abs

A "spare tire" around your waistline is a definite problem. Unwanted fat, especially at your midsection, increases your risk of diabetes, heart disease, high blood pressure, and some cancers. A recent study finds it can lead to lung problems, as well.

Naturally, you want to do something about it, but are gut-wrenching sit-ups the best way to get rid of a fat belly? Not according to Dr. Bryant Stamford, a professor of physiology at the University of Louisville, Ky. Writing in *The Physician And Sportsmedicine*, he points out there is no such thing as spot reduction. When you exercise, you don't necessarily burn fat from around the muscles you are using. If you want to get the most out of your abdominal workout, follow these tips.

Use your mind to keep your body fit

Thinking of your daily activities as exercise can actually give you a great workout. That's what two Harvard psychologists found when they studied hotel housekeepers. The researchers focused on 84 women who typically clean 15 hotel rooms each day, taking 20 to 30 minutes for each room. Some of the women viewed a presentation explaining that their strenuous jobs provide good exercise and fit the guidelines for a healthy lifestyle. The other women were told nothing.

Although none of the housekeepers changed what they were doing, those who believed they were getting exercise had better health after just four weeks. In fact, they lost an average of two pounds each, lowered their blood pressure, and reduced their body mass index (BMI). In contrast, the women who were not told their jobs counted as exercise showed no health changes.

Burn more calories. The fat you burn when you exercise may come from anywhere on your body, so Stamford recommends doing the activities that use the most calories. He says you'd have to do hundreds of sit-ups to equal the calories you'd burn on a brisk walk or jog.

Relax to stay trim. Exercise may be necessary for removing your potbelly, but reducing stress can help keep it off. For some reason, stress releases chemicals that cause fat to shift from other parts of your body to your waistline. Listening to music, meditating, or talking to a friend or counselor about your problems can help relieve stress. These practices also help you keep a positive attitude, which makes it easier to stick to your diet and exercise plan.

Tighten muscles for a sharper shape. Suck in your stomach when exercising, because a bouncing belly weakens the abdominal muscles. And don't forget to stretch your hamstrings. Strengthening these muscles on the back of your thighs helps prevent a swayback, which can make your stomach stick out even more.

Although they won't remove the fat, sit-ups can strengthen your abdominal muscles and protect your back. If full sit-ups seem too difficult, do just the second half, where you lower yourself down. Here's how:

▶ Starting from a sitting position with hands at your sides, place your feet flat on the floor with your legs at a 90-degree angle. This way your abdominal muscles, not your legs and hips, will do the work.

▶ Tense your belly and slowly – so your muscles work against gravity's downward pull – lower yourself until your back touches the floor.

▶ Push yourself back up with your arms.

▶ Repeat five times at first, adding a few more each time you work out.

To exercise your abdominal muscles a little harder, increase resistance by crossing your arms over your chest.

Weight-loss secret you can't do without

Walking doesn't require any special talent or training – you do it naturally without thinking. Yet, if you put a little extra time and effort into it each day, just look at the results. You lose weight, have more energy, avoid diabetes, lower your blood pressure and cholesterol, think more clearly, have less anxiety, and sleep a whole lot better. And that's just the beginning.

Benefits like these have turned walking into one of the most popular fitness activities ever. People tend to give up on most exercise programs after the first big push, but walkers are more like the Energizer Bunny – they just keep on going. That's because they discover it is a steady, sure way to health and fitness. They don't stop when they get older, either. More men over age 65 are regular walkers than in any other age group. For many people, a daily walk has become their ticket to a longer, healthier, more enjoyable life.

A daily walk of 30 minutes or more is the weight-loss secret you can't do without. Do you know the magic number? Remember 10,000. That's the number of steps you should aim for each day to lower your body fat and weight, get a slimmer waist and hips, lower your blood pressure, improve your glucose control, and increase your "good" cholesterol. Most people who don't exercise take about 5,000 steps per day, so you'll have to find ways to get moving. An inexpensive step counter can help you keep track of your progress.

Want more reasons to walk? Try these and see if they don't persuade you to put on your walking shoes right now.

Smart way to keep blood sugar stable

Exercise is a great way to lose weight and keep your diabetes under control. But if you have diabetes, you need to test your blood sugar level before and after you exercise. As you work out, your body's cells take in sugar to use for energy. That makes your blood sugar level drop. Some people find eating a small snack before an exercise session helps keep blood sugar stable. Ask your doctor about adjusting your drugs to compensate for physical activity.

▶ Walking is just as good as running for burning excess calories and helping to control diabetes. The fact is, you burn just as many calories per mile walking as you do running. It just takes longer – 20 minutes to walk a mile versus eight or 10 minutes to jog it. Be sure to walk briskly. You won't experience much conditioning or weight loss unless you raise your heart rate.

▶ You can walk just about any time you're in the mood. You don't have to make a reservation, change clothes, or wait for others to join you.

▶ You're less likely to get hurt than with other activities. Walking is low impact, so you don't have the stress on your joints that leads to blown-out knees, sprained ankles, and bad backs. Other health risks are almost zero because it's less strenuous than most activities.

▶ You can afford it. There are no clubs to join or expensive equipment to buy. All you really need is a pair of sturdy shoes. Just dust off your old sneakers – or better yet invest in a new pair – and get up and go.

▶ You can do it anywhere – in your own neighborhood or local park, while you're shopping, even when you're out-of-town. If the weather is bad, walk indoors.

Make a commitment. Walking won't help much if you don't do it regularly, so find the motivation to stick with it. Come up with reasons why exercising is important to you. Perhaps you want to wear attractive styles of clothing, or maybe you want to be able to keep up with your grandchildren. Write down your own reasons, and put the list on your refrigerator to remind you why walking is important to you. To get through the first few weeks, tell your plans to family and friends. You'll be embarrassed if you don't follow through, and they can encourage you and praise your progress.

Decide on a time. Once you've decided why you're going to walk, decide when – every morning, every evening, every other afternoon – and write it down on your calendar. You may have to make some choices, like cutting out a half hour of TV or getting up an hour earlier in the morning. But scheduling exercise in writing shows you're serious about fitting it into your daily life.

Pick your place. Where should you walk? Anywhere your heart desires. That's the beauty of this type of exercise. Of course, you want to make sure it's a safe area, and pleasant surroundings wouldn't hurt, either.

If you prefer the outdoors, you can walk on streets and sidewalks, in parks, or on trails built especially for walking. If you want a smooth, level surface, look for a school with an athletic track. In cities like Reston, Va., and Peachtree City, Ga., golf carts are a way of life, and you can walk on miles and miles of cart paths. Some places also have bicycle trails you can use.

Add some fun to your walks

Hate exercise? That's OK. You can do this — go for a walk. Whether you have trouble crossing the room, or you're walking a few miles a day, these tips will help get you moving.

▸ Have a destination, such as a coffee shop, post office, or library.

▸ Go where you can enjoy window-shopping while you walk.

▸ Use your time for planning your day or just relaxing and thinking.

▸ Take along your dog, someone else's dog, or a friend or family member for company.

▸ Choose alternate routes each day. Get adventurous and explore new neighborhoods.

Be careful when you share space with vehicles. Remember, it's hard for cars to avoid people in the street, and it's hard to hear golf carts and bicycles coming up behind you. To walk indoors, go to large stores or shopping malls, or use the treadmills at gyms and other athletic facilities. You can even go from room to room in your own home.

Before long, you'll be keeping up with the best of walkers and reaping the benefits of the walking fitness phenomenon.

Stretch the benefits of exercise

Stretching is the Rodney Dangerfield of the exercise world. It gets no respect. You may think stretching is only something you're supposed to do before you play a sport. Worse, you may not stretch at all because you think it's not important. That's a shame for your body. Stretching is a crucial part of fitness. It helps you get the most from walking, strength training, golf, or whatever other activities you enjoy. On top of that, it's worth doing for its own sake. The more flexible you are, the easier and more pleasant your everyday activities will be.

It's natural to be less flexible as you age, but stretching is a natural way to slow and even reverse this process. When you include it in your exercise regimen, you'll quickly notice the improvements. You may become flexible enough to sit on the floor and play with your grandkids. Or you may be able to reach for groceries high up on the supermarket shelf without any help. Consider these stretching benefits:

▶ Your muscles will return to their full range of motion. That may lead to balance and coordination you haven't had for decades, which could reduce your danger of sudden falls or slips. Flexible, fit muscles also mean better posture and fewer everyday aches and pains.

▶ Your blood may flow better if you stretch. More nutrients will reach your muscles, while waste products will be flushed away.

▶ A stretched muscle may be at less risk for injury. If your muscle is already injured, stretching could help reduce healing time.

▶ It helps loosen those knots left behind by the daily grind, just like giving yourself a massage.

Before you get started, here are a few suggestions to help you get the most from your stretching routine.

Warm up before you stretch. You wouldn't jump into the shower right after turning on the water. The cold water would shock your system. Instead, you'd wait for the water to warm up. Same thing for stretching. Don't dive right in when your muscles are still cold. Spend several minutes warming them up by doing jumping jacks, riding a real or stationary bike, walking while pumping your arms, or running in place. Any of these can get your heart rate up, loosen your muscles and joints, and prepare you for an injury-free workout.

Work slowly and gently. It's best to stretch all your major muscle groups any time you do a stretching routine. In other words, loosen all the muscles you usually use – your legs, back, neck, and other upper-body muscles. If you're in a rush, however, loosen only the muscles you need at the moment. Work on your legs before you jog, or stretch your shoulders before you golf. Afterward, make sure to do a complete stretch.

For all your muscles, follow these easy stretching guidelines.

▶ Reach as far as you can. Don't feel you have to touch your toes or bend over backward. For any stretch, reach until you feel a slight tension in your muscle. If you feel pain or a burning sensation, you've gone too deep. Ease back until the pain goes away.

▶ Hold it for at least 30 seconds. Do each stretch for this long, and you'll only need to do it once. A whole minute may be needed if your muscle is really tight. Time yourself with a stopwatch at

Clamp down on muscle cramps

Experts at the American Academy of Orthopaedic Surgeons say tight muscles may have a lot to do with cramps. Stretching seems to get at the root of cramp problems, they suggest, because it lengthens and loosens muscle fibers. That's great news for seniors, since cramps are a major pain in the neck or leg for many.

During a bout of calf cramps, try stretching the tight muscle by straightening your leg and bending your foot up toward your shin. If you can stand, put your weight on the aching leg and bend your knee a little. Massaging a cramped muscle can help, too.

Dehydration can also bring on muscle cramps. If you're active, take in at least six to eight glasses of water a day. However, cramping may have more serious causes. If stretching and refueling on fluids don't do the trick, talk to your doctor.

first to get the feel of how long this is. If you really enjoy stretching and feel you need it, repeat each stretch three to five times.

▶ Feel at ease and breathe. This session is not a workout for your lungs, so breathe normally. You're not supposed to clench your muscles, either. Relax every muscle except the ones you're stretching at the moment.

▶ Do not bounce. No matter what your gym teacher taught you in high school, do not bounce when you stretch. You risk injury by bouncing, and it may even make you less flexible.

Whether you're young or young at heart, active or wishing you were, stretching is a great way to get in shape.

Quick and easy way to get fit

Regular, low-impact aerobic exercise lets you reap big rewards with relatively little time and effort – especially if you've been a couch potato. All forms of this type of exercise concentrate on fitness and endurance more than strength. If you stick to low-impact activities, which don't cause jarring and strain on your joints, there's less wear and tear on your body.

People with diabetes get extra gains from aerobic exercise. Regular moderate aerobic activity may help control your blood sugar by improving insulin sensitivity. It also protects against heart disease and helps control your weight.

By definition, aerobic exercise uses the oxygen you breathe to produce energy and allows you to work out for a long period of time. Aerobic activities include jogging, dancing, bicycling, skating, swimming, and even shoveling and mowing.

Walking is the quickest and easiest way to start an aerobic program. However, if you're looking for greater variety or a bigger challenge, there are plenty of other fun aerobic exercises you can do. Some, like bicycling yourself into shape for a road race, involve pushing yourself harder and farther. Others, like water and step aerobics, might mean enrolling in a class. But all aerobic activities will improve your overall fitness.

Strengthen your heart and lungs. An aerobic exercise raises your heart rate and keeps it up at around 60 to 85 percent of your heart rate maximum. This increases the amount of oxygen your body delivers to your muscles. The more oxygen they have, the longer they can work without fatiguing. Therefore, aerobic exercise strengthens your heart and increases your lungs' ability to gather oxygen, making the whole system more efficient.

Good aerobic activity is continuous, repetitive, and usually rhythmic. It works large muscles at a pace that uses oxygen about as fast as you take it in. When this happens, you give your muscles a constant bath of fresh oxygen while your heart and lungs get a good workout. As they become stronger, you can exercise longer and harder with less effort. The result — you gain endurance and muscle tone.

Burn away fat. Aerobic exercise is great for weight loss, too. It speeds up your metabolism, which stimulates the fat-burning process. Your metabolism continues at a faster pace even after you've stopped exercising, which means you burn more fat.

Reduce stress on joints. The water is a terrific place for fitness. Its buoyancy reduces the stress on your weight-bearing joints by as much as 90 percent, cutting down on muscle soreness and injury. Yet, water provides the resistance needed to develop a strong heart and lungs.

To bebop or cha-cha — that's the question

If you'd like to dance your way to fitness, ask yourself these questions to help you decide which style of dance to try.

▸ What kind of music do you enjoy? If you like country songs, zydeco, or bluegrass music, square dancing may be for you. If you love music from past decades or Latin music, you might try ballroom dance.

▸ Would you rather dance alone, with a partner, or as part of a group? Ballroom dance requires a partner, but you can participate in any line dance without one.

▸ Are classes available in your area, or can you be happy learning from a video? A local hula instructor may be tough to find.

▸ What type of dance have you always dreamed of trying? If you're motivated by a true love of dance, you'll be more inclined to stick with it.

Water aerobics is probably the ultimate low-impact exercise. It's sometimes the only way for certain people to exercise — people with arthritis, the elderly, people who are overweight, or those recovering from surgery or injury. But anyone can benefit.

The best way to take advantage of water aerobics, even if you have your own pool, is to enroll in a class. You can find one through local recreation departments, the YMCA or YWCA, or health clubs and gyms. In water aerobics classes, you'll spend about 10 minutes stretching, and then you'll work with belts, ankle straps, and light-weight dumbbells that serve as both flotation and resistance devices. You'll also walk and run in the water and do exercises while suspended in the water.

Improve flexibility and muscle tone. If a bit of the old soft shoe is not in your current game plan, rethink your strategy. Dancing can be a great aerobic exercise that improves flexibility and tones muscles. It's also a weight-bearing activity good for anyone concerned about bone loss from osteoporosis. Although dance can have aerobic benefits, you don't need to wear yourself out. Any form of dance can be slowed down to make it less demanding. In general, dance is good for cardiovascular fitness, strength, endurance, and flexibility. A dance class also lets you be social while you're getting fit.

You can get aerobic exercise from activities other than walking, water aerobics, swimming, or dancing. Most require special settings and equipment, but all have an element of excitement. If you like being around water, try rowing or canoeing — you can even take along a fishing pole. If you live where there's snow, cross-country skiing and snowshoeing are better exercise than walking. Ice-skating or roller-skating can be fun if you don't have balance problems.

Jogging and jumping rope are higher impact ways to get your heart beating. Athletics, like handball, racquetball, basketball, and soccer, also provide good workouts.

Burn more calories with strength training

You don't have to be Charles Atlas to power up with strength training. This kind of exercise is a key to fitness for everyone – especially seniors. Stacks of scientific studies prove this. In fact, senior muscles may benefit from strength training more than young ones. Strength training has many names. Resistance training, weight lifting, working out, and pumping iron are just a few. Whatever you call it, it's more valuable, easy, and fun than you probably imagined.

For instance, you may not know strength training can rev up your metabolism and help you burn more calories around the clock. It gets results by stressing your muscles more than your humdrum daily activities do. This stress could come from doing pushups, pressing a dumbbell above your head, or curling a coffee can. Believe it or not, muscles live for this extra work. It makes them stronger and healthier.

Strike a blow against diabetes. Surprisingly, you may enjoy some of the most dramatic benefits from strength training if you have type 2 diabetes. It could help you get a grip on blood sugar control, according to an Australian study of overweight people with diabetes ages 60 to 80.

In this study, one group of men and women lifted weights three days a week for six months while eating a healthy, low-calorie diet. Another group ate the wholesome diet and did stretching exercises. Both groups lost weight at the end of the research, but only the strength-training seniors gained lean body mass and significantly improved their blood sugar control.

The scientists Down Under were not sure exactly how it worked. They suspected muscle works like a blood-sugar sponge, absorbing glucose out of your system. The strength-training group gained muscle mass as their blood sugar dropped. The second group, on the other hand, lost some of their muscle mass. So this theory seems to make sense.

As all people with diabetes know, better blood sugar control means fewer side effects, like heart disease, nerve and kidney problems, and blindness. You don't need more reasons than these to start pumping iron. But remember, check with your doctor before you head for the gym.

Put the brakes on aging. You lose as much as 40 percent of your muscle strength during your adult life, health experts say. This process — called sarcopenia — starts in your 40s and 50s, when your muscle fibers begin to shrink, become less efficient, and disappear altogether. Sarcopenia leads to the weakness, poor coordination, and bad balance that many seniors suffer. Strength training halts this process and may even reverse it. According to the latest research, your strength could jump by an amazing 100 percent if you're a weight-lifting senior. Pumping iron works because it encourages your muscles to grow and become more responsive and powerful.

Lifting weights can also build up your bones. When muscles flex during strength training, the bones around them respond like plants to sunlight — they grow. And it doesn't matter how old you are when you start. Even seniors with osteoporosis can benefit from low-weight, high-rep resistance training.

When you follow a regular lifting program, you'll see muscles you haven't noticed since you were 30 years old. Strength training carves muscles until they become lean and well-defined. Moreover, extra muscle helps protect your joints and lower back during aerobic exercises, such as jogging and bicycling.

Master the rules to achieve your goals. Every strength-training exercise has its own stance and movements, which you'll find pictured on pages 315-324. Before you grasp those, it's important to master these universal rules. They can help you prevent injury no matter which exercise you do.

▶ Practice good posture. Always stand or sit straight. Keep your chin in and lined up with your neck and back. Unlock your knees and leave them loose. If you're seated, angle your knees at 90 degrees.

▸ Relax. Let your body be loose. Allow your shoulders to hang in their natural position. Tense only the particular muscle you're exercising at the time.

▸ Slow down. Whether the exercise calls for you to push or pull, move the weights and your muscles slowly. As a rough guide, take two to three seconds to do an exercise's flexing motion. Hold it for a second. Then spend four to five seconds returning to the starting position.

Get fit without really trying

Exercise helps control your weight and lower your risk for diabetes. It's never too early or too late to get started. Statistics show if you are overweight when you are 25, you are more likely to have diabetes in middle age. Adding exercise to your daily routine need not be a burden. Try these simple suggestions.

▸ Park farther away in parking lots.

▸ Walk while you're on the telephone and during TV commercials.

▸ Go inside a restaurant instead of using the drive-through.

▸ Take the stairs instead of the elevator.

▸ Take a walk with family or friends in a garden or park.

▸ Go bowling with friends or family.

▸ Lift hand-held weights as you talk on the phone.

▸ Rock in a rocking chair.

▸ Dance as you perform household chores.

▶ Concentrate. Never jerk, swing, or bounce a dumbbell or bar-bell. That's one way injuries occur. Always have control over the weight, and stay within a comfortable range of motion. If you can't, you may be tired. Stop and rest for the next set.

▶ Breathe. Sounds simple enough, but if you don't breathe while you work out, your blood pressure could shoot through the roof. Most experts recommend exhaling while you contract your mus-cle and inhaling when you relax. But don't think too hard about it — just breathe like you normally would.

▶ Take a day off. Listen to your body. Pass on exercise when you feel under-the-weather, tired, or overly sore. Working out then may only make you feel worse.

Gentle way to increase strength and flexibility

The gentle practice of yoga is an ancient art with great benefits for modern people. Yoga is an easy way to lose weight and rejuvenate your metabolism. When your metabolism is revved up, you auto-matically burn more fat.

The yoga approach to weight loss involves both physical and mental exercises — boosting your self-confidence and strengthening your self-control.

You may not think yoga is strenuous enough to help you lose weight, but it's a lot more challenging than it looks. This ancient art helps you build strength and flexibility and works on your aerobic conditioning, breathing, and relaxation.

In fact, this total body-mind focus is the key to its success in weight management. By embracing the "holistic" mindset of all-around good health, including reaching and maintaining a healthy weight, you incorporate a positive attitude into all aspects of your life.

Yoga is a program that helps you cultivate realistic goals and expectations, rather than a get-thin-quick mindset that focuses on killer exercises and fad dieting. It helps you understand why you're overweight and provides a means of addressing those issues through exercise and relaxation.

The traditional poses can be done at your own pace, either alone or with a group, and this benefit is an incentive to stick with the program. The deep breathing and slow movements help relieve stress and provide you with renewed energy. Once you incorporate yoga into your life, you'll wonder how you ever managed without it. See pages 325-327 for some basic yoga moves to get you started.

A study conducted by the University of Pittsburgh shows yoga can help you lose weight. A group of 59 obese, inactive women were placed on a low-fat diet and assigned to either walk, walk and do strength-training exercises, or walk and do yoga.

After four months, those who only walked lost an average of 20 pounds. Those who walked and did strength-training exercises lost an average of 23 pounds. And those who walked and did yoga lost an average of 27 pounds.

Age gracefully with tai chi

Originally developed as a martial arts style of self-defense, tai chi uses a series of postures and slow, continuous movements to relax and align your body. Through the years, it has become a form of exercise with many benefits.

▶ Improves your balance. It teaches you to be aware of your surroundings and boosts your muscle tone. Better balance means fewer falls. In fact, tai chi can reduce your risk of falling by almost 50 percent.

▶ Relaxes your heart and your mind. Seniors who practiced tai chi 30 minutes a day, four days a week for 12 weeks, reduced their blood pressure about as much as those in a more strenuous aerobic exercise program. Tai chi can also relieve stress and boost your memory.

▸ Eases arthritis pain. Dr. Paul Lam, a medical doctor and student of tai chi for more than 30 years, is a world leader in the field of tai chi for health improvement. He has developed a special program called Tai Chi for Arthritis.

You don't need expensive equipment to try tai chi, but wear comfortable shoes and loose clothing. A little knowledge can get you started right.

A full set of tai chi exercises is called a form. The basic short form has 37 different moves. It can take up to a year to learn the whole form. But don't worry about an entire form. Stay focused on the move you are in and not the one up ahead. Don't move on until you get it right. It's more important to practice tai chi every day than to learn the moves quickly.

While doing tai chi movements, be sure to control your weight shifts. This means when you move, you first shift all your weight onto your supporting leg. Next, place your other foot, and only then move your weight to that leg. This will help you move smoothly. Remember, tai chi should look fluid — not robotic.

To get into the correct starting position for tai chi, stand with your feet shoulder-width apart, toes pointed forward. Bend your knees just slightly so you drop down about 2 inches. Don't lean, but distribute your weight evenly. Keep your upper body straight, your head and shoulders relaxed, and your hands loose at your sides. Stand like this for two to three minutes.

Anxious to try out a bit of tai chi? See pages 328-330 for a few moves to whet your appetite. You may see tai chi practiced on beaches and in parks in your area. Join in if you're comfortable with the whole form.

Stretch and strengthen with Pilates

In the early 1900s, Joseph Pilates developed a new form of physical therapy that combined Eastern and Western ideas about fitness. Borrowing from yoga and the gymnastics of ancient Greek and Roman regimens, it focuses on stretching and lengthening the muscles, along with improving posture. At the core of his program are six principles – breath, concentration, control, centering, precision, and flow. Strict Pilates is a combination of mat work and machine-aided exercises. The mat work is easy to learn and can be practiced anywhere. The movements are slow, graceful, and – best of all – low-impact. They are so effective, you can forget traditional sit-ups. These exercises will even flatten a bulging belly and strengthen your back, while improving your posture and balance.

Of the three movement therapies, Pilates is the most physically demanding, vigorous enough to qualify as a strength-training program. And you'll see speedy results. Many people notice a difference after just 10 to 20 sessions. When combined with a cardiovascular exercise, like walking or swimming, Pilates is a full-body fitness program.

As the name suggests, all you need for the Pilates mat work is a good exercise mat and comfortable clothing. Socks or bare feet work best. Follow these tips to get the most from your workout.

▸ Keep your tummy tucked in while doing Pilates moves. Draw the muscles in your abdomen toward your spine, sort of like pulling in to zip up tight pants. If you tighten your lower back and buttocks muscles at the same time, the movement is called engaging your powerhouse.

▸ Stand with your feet in a V shape, with heels together and toes slightly open. Squeeze your buttocks and thighs together. This will twist your calves out slightly. The position is actually the same even if you're lying down and your feet are in the air.

▸ Keep a bit of space between your chin and chest when you're told to lift your head off the mat, and always look straight ahead. If this is difficult, you can leave your head down, or prop it on a towel or cushion.

▶ Don't hold your breath during any exercise. Keep breathing deeply the entire time, in through your nose and out through your mouth.

▶ Concentrate fully on each motion. Focus on your body — lengthening muscles and maintaining good posture.

Not sure about the moves? Consider a session with a trained Pilates instructor. She can explain the machines and make sure you're using proper form so you don't get hurt.

Begin with five simple Pilates exercises to help you banish an unsightly belly and give you leaner abdominal muscles. See pages 331-334 for details.

LEGS Hamstring stretch

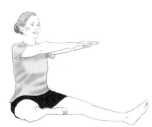

1. Sit up on the floor or in your bed.
2. Extend your left leg. Fold in your right leg so its foot points toward your right knee.
3. Lean forward, reaching your arms above your legs and leaving your back straight. Don't overreach to touch your toes. Hold for 15 to 20 seconds.
4. Extend your right leg, fold your left, and repeat.

LEGS Butterfly stretch

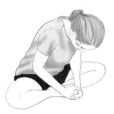

1. Sit with your feet touching in front of you.
2. Hold your feet, leaning your elbows into the inside of your knees.
3. Push down gently on your knees until you feel a stretch in your groin. Hold for 5 seconds.

LEGS Thigh stretch

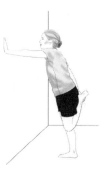

1. Stand facing a wall at arm's length. Place your left hand on it for support.

2. Lift up your left foot behind you, and grab it with your right hand.

3. Pull your left foot toward your buttocks, and hold for 30 seconds.

4. Let go of your left foot, switch hands and feet, and repeat with your right leg.

LEGS Calf stretch

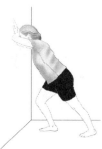

1. Stand about a foot away from a wall. Lean against it with your forearms, and rest your head on your hands.

2. Step forward with your right foot, bending that leg. Keep your left leg straight.

3. Lean forward until you feel a tug in the back of your left leg. Hold for 15 to 30 seconds.

4. Switch legs and repeat.

BACK Knee-to-chest stretch

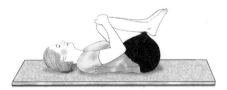

1. Lie on your back on the floor or in your bed.

2. Fold your legs on top of you so your knees touch your chest.

3. Grab your knees, and pull them down until you feel a stretch in your lower back. Hold for 30 seconds.

BACK Pelvic tilt

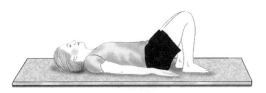

1. Lie on your back on the floor or in your bed.

2. Bend your knees, and plant your feet about one foot away from your buttocks.

3. Press the small of your back toward the floor, and tighten your abdominal muscles. Use your hips, not your legs. Hold for 5 seconds, then relax.

NECK Head tilt

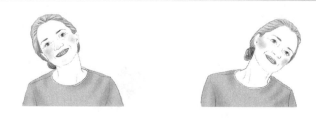

1. Sit up in a chair or in your bed.

2. Look straight ahead. Relax your shoulders.

3. Tilt your head to the right, leaning your ear toward your shoulder. When you feel a gentle stretch in your neck, hold for 10 seconds.

4. Straighten your head, then repeat to the left side.

NECK Shoulder roll

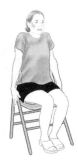

1. Sit in a chair or your bed with your arms at your sides.

2. Shrug your shoulders upward without bending your elbows.

3. Rotate your shoulders forward in a circle. Then rotate them backward.

4. Repeat each direction at least five times, making each circle bigger than the last.

UPPER BODY Over-the-head shoulder stretch

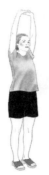

1. Stand up, or sit up in a chair or in bed.

2. Reach your arms over your head as far as they can go, and interlace your fingers.

3. Turn your palms upward. Gently push your arms back and up. Hold for 15 seconds.

UPPER BODY Upper body twist

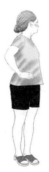

1. Stand up and place your hands on your hips.

2. Twist your upper body to the left as far as it can go, leaving your legs facing forward. Hold for 5 seconds.

3. Repeat to the right.

CHEST Arm twist

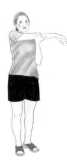

1. Sit or stand up.

2. Reach your right arm across your chest in front of your left shoulder.

3. Place your left hand on your right elbow and gently push. You'll feel a stretch in the back of your shoulder. Hold.

4. Switch arms and repeat.

CHEST Shoulder rotation

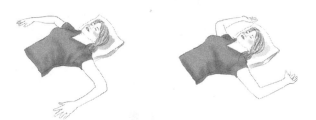

1. Lie on the floor or in your bed with a pillow beneath your head. If you have back problems, put a rolled towel underneath your knees.

2. Lay your arms out perpendicular to your body, and bend them up at the elbows so they look like goalposts.

3. Rotate your arms forward, moving your hands to the floor near your waist. Hold for 20 to 30 seconds.

4. Rotate your forearms up and then backward, moving your hands toward the floor near your head. Hold.

CHEST Wall press

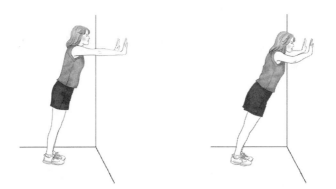

1. Stand facing a wall at arms' length.

2. Place both of your hands against the wall at shoulder height.

3. Bend your elbows, and slowly lower your chest toward the wall.

4. Push yourself back up to finish the rep.

CHEST Modified knee push-up

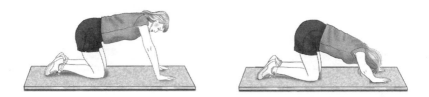

1. Get down on your hands and knees.

2. Lay your hands on the floor below but slightly ahead of your shoulders.

3. Bend your elbows, and lower your chest as close to the ground as possible.

4. Push yourself back up to end the rep.

BACK One-arm dumbbell row

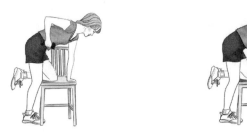

1. Stand to the right of a chair or flat bench. Place a dumbbell on the floor to the chair's right.

2. Rest your left knee on the chair, lean forward, and plant your left hand on the chair. Grab the dumbbell with your right hand.

3. Keeping your back parallel to the chair, pull the weight up toward your chest.

4. Lower the weight to end the rep. After 10 to 15 reps, switch and work your left arm.

BACK Back extension

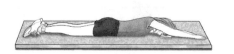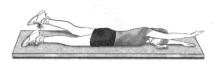

1. Lie face down on your stomach with your legs and arms extended.

2. Fold a towel under your forehead for padding.

3. Lift your right arm and left leg a few inches off the ground. Tighten your stomach muscles while lifting.

4. Lower them, and repeat with the opposite arm and leg to finish the rep.

BACK/SHOULDERS Shoulder shrug

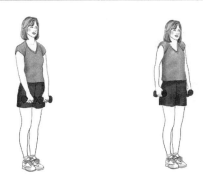

1. Stand with a dumbbell in each hand.

2. Rest them on the sides of your legs with your knuckles out.

3. Pull your shoulders up toward your ears, leaving your arms straight.

4. Lower them back down to end the rep.

BACK/SHOULDERS Upward row

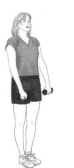 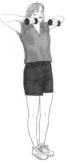

1. Stand holding a dumbbell in each hand.

2. Let your arms hang down with the weights in front of your body and your knuckles out.

3. Move the weights toward your chin by pulling your hands straight up.

4. Stop at shoulder height, and lower the weights back down to finish the rep.

LEGS No-weight squat

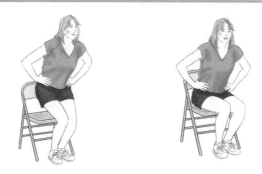

1. Sit on a sturdy chair or flat bench.

2. Hold your hands on your hips for balance.

3. Lean forward and stand up, keeping your body centered over your feet.

4. Sit back down to end the rep.

LEGS Lunge

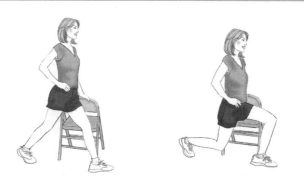

1. Stand to the right of a sturdy chair, which you can hold for support.

2. Set your feet about three feet apart, with your left foot forward and your right foot in back.

3. Bend both knees and lower your body straight down. Don't allow your front knee to go past your toe.

4. Push back up and stand to end the rep. After 10 to 15 reps, switch leg positions and repeat.

LEGS Back leg swing

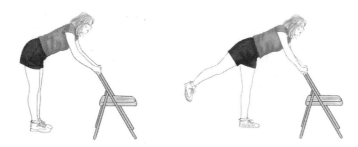

1. Stand one to two feet behind a sturdy chair.

2. Bend at the waist and lean forward, supporting yourself on the back of the chair.

3. Raise your right leg straight behind you until it's in line with your back.

4. Return your foot to the floor to end the rep. After 10 to 15 reps with your right leg, switch to your left.

LEGS Side leg swing

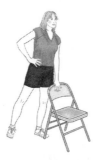

1. Stand behind a sturdy chair, and hold the back for balance.

2. Slowly lift your right leg straight out to the side until it's 6 inches off the ground.

3. Lower your foot to the floor to end the rep. After 10 to 15 reps, switch to your left leg and repeat.

319

Strength training

LEGS Calf raise

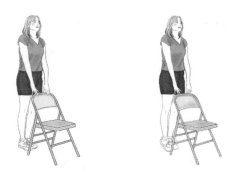

1. Stand behind a sturdy chair, and hold on to the back for balance.

2. Push up with your toes, and lift both heels off the floor.

3. Slowly lower back down to end the rep.

SHOULDERS Military press

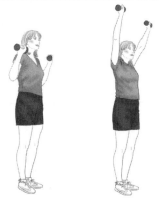

1. Stand with a dumbbell in each hand.

2. Raise the weights to your shoulders. Keep your arms below your shoulders with your elbows bent and your palms facing forward.

3. Push the dumbbells above your head until your arms are straight. Don't arch your back.

4. Lower the weights to your shoulders to end the rep.

SHOULDERS Lateral dumbbell raise

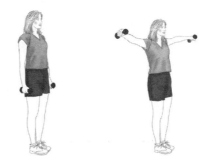

1. Stand with a dumbbell in each hand.

2. Rest them on the sides of your hips with your knuckles out.

3. Slowly raise your arms out to the sides, keeping your elbows slightly bent.

4. Stop at shoulder height, and lower them back down to finish the rep.

SHOULDERS Front dumbbell raise

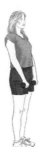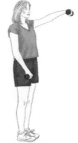

1. Stand with a dumbbell in each hand.

2. Rest them on the front of your thighs with your knuckles out.

3. Slowly raise your left arm in front of you, keeping your elbows slightly bent.

4. Stop at shoulder height, and lower it back down. Raise and lower your right arm to end the rep.

ARMS Bicep curl

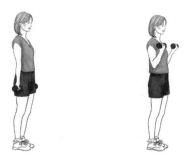

1. Pick up a dumbbell in each hand. Let your arms hang down with the weights at your sides and your palms facing forward.

2. Bend at your elbows, and pull the weights up toward your shoulders. Move only your forearms — not your upper arms.

3. Lower your forearms back down to your sides to complete the rep.

ARMS Overhead tricep extension

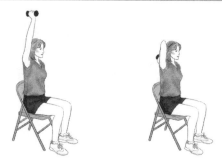

1. Sit with a dumbbell in your right hand. Hold the weight over your head.

2. Bend your right elbow, and slowly lower the dumbbell toward your shoulder. Keep your elbow near your ear, pointing forward. Use your left hand to support your arm, if needed.

3. Slowly straighten your arm, and press the weight above your head. After 10 to 15 reps, switch arms and repeat.

ARMS Tricep kickback

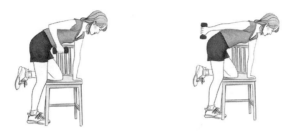

1. Place a dumbbell on a chair or flat bench. Standing to the right of the chair, rest your left knee on it and lean forward over the weight.

2. Place your left hand on the bench. Pick up the dumbbell with your right hand. Cock your elbow back so your arm makes an L. Keep your back straight.

3. Straighten your right arm, pushing the weight backward. Only your fore-arm should move — not your whole arm.

4. Lower your forearm back into the L position to finish the rep. After 10 to 15 reps with your right arm, repeat with your left.

ABS Abdominal press

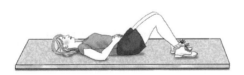

1. Lie on the floor or bed on your back.

2. Bend your knees, and plant your feet on the floor.

3. Flatten the small of your back against the floor using your stomach muscles.

4. Hold. Relax to end the rep.

ABS Leg lift

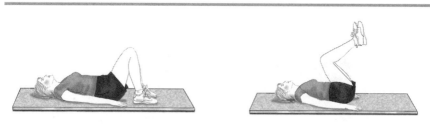

1. Lie on the floor on your back.
   Bend your knees, and plant your feet on the floor a foot or two from your buttocks.

2. Lift your legs off the ground, and bring your thighs as close to your ribs as possible. Squeeze your abdominals.

3. Lower your legs so they almost touch the ground to complete one rep.

ABS Crunch

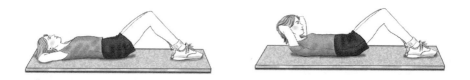

1. Lie on the floor on your back. Fold your hands behind your head.

2. Bend your knees, and plant your feet on the floor about a foot from your buttocks.

3. Lift your head, shoulders, and upper back off the ground using your stomach muscles — not your arms.

4. Lower yourself to the ground to end the rep.

Yoga Mountain pose

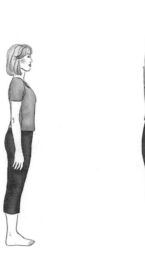

1. Stand tall, your feet together, your hands at your sides, and your weight evenly balanced.

2. Spread your toes apart and settle your feet firmly onto the floor.

3. Tuck you hips in, and puff your chest out just a bit.

4. Lengthen your neck by lifting the top of your head toward the ceiling.

5. Imagine a line running straight up through your body and out the top of your head.

6. Hold this pose for 5 to 10 slow, deep breaths.

7. Raise your arms over your head with your palms inward.

8. Breathe in deeply. Imagine the air coming up through your body, then going back down to your toes. Hold this pose for 5 to 10 breaths.

9. Lower your arms on an exhale and repeat 5 times.

Yoga Easy cobra lift

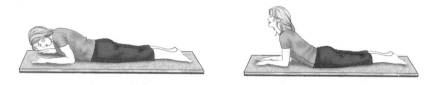

1. Lie down on your stomach. Place your elbows on the mat close to your body, and your palms flat on the mat near your head.

2. Without lifting your elbows off the floor, raise your chest up and out. Keep your hips and legs flat against the mat.

3. Don't tilt your head too far back. Look ahead and hold the pose for a few seconds.

4. Release, relax, and repeat twice more.

Yoga Child's pose

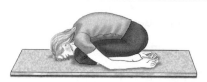

1. Assume a kneeling position with the tops of your feet against your mat.

2. Lower your buttocks down until they rest on your heels. If you have difficulty with this position, place a folded blanket between your calves and your buttocks.

3. Bend forward and drop your chest onto your thighs.

4. Relax your shoulders and rest your forehead gently on the mat or on a pillow.

5. Drape your arms loosely at your sides, palms up.

6. Relax, breathing deeply.

7. Hold for a minute or two.

8. Return very slowly to a sitting position.

Yoga Half warrior

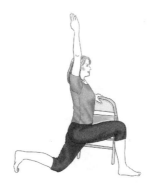

1. Place your right foot 3 to 4 feet in front of your body.

2. Drop your left knee gently to the floor so you are in a lunge position. Keep your right knee in line with your right ankle.

3. If you need to, hold on to a chair or table for balance, or place a blanket under your knee.

4. Keeping your back straight and your eyes forward, inhale and bring your arms straight up over your head. Place your palms together.

5. Hold for 4 or 5 deep breaths, then return to your starting position.

6. Repeat on the other side.

Tai Chi

Tai Chi Swimming in deep water

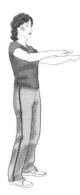 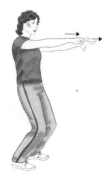 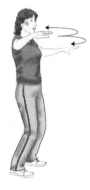

1. Stand with your knees slightly bent. Raise your hands to chest height, palms down, elbows slightly bent.

2. Breathe in.

3. Imagine you're about to swim the breast stroke.

4. Gently extend your arms forward.

5. Sink lower into your knees and breathe out.

6. Keep your back straight, your head up, and your eyes looking forward.

7. Finish the breast-stroke movement by drawing your arms back, in a flat, outward circle. Breathe in.

8. At the same time, straighten slightly to your previous position.

9. Repeat 10 to 30 times.

Tai Chi Working the oar

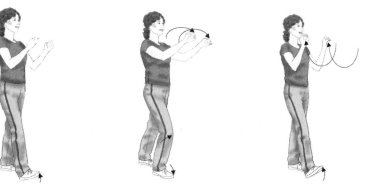

1. Start with your feet about shoulder-width apart. Shift your weight to your left leg.

2. Move your right foot about a foot forward.

3. Raise your hands to chest height, elbows down, and pretend you are holding oars in your hands.

4. Breathe in.

5. Smoothly shift your weight completely onto your right leg. Keep your knee behind the line of your toes.

6. As you breathe out, extend your arms in a forward and downward circular motion, as though rowing.

7. Shift your weight gradually back onto your left foot, lifting the front of your right foot off the floor. Breathe in.

8. Bring your hands back toward your chest to your starting position.

9. Practice this move about 30 times with the right foot forward, then 30 times with the left.

Tai Chi Showing your palms and soles

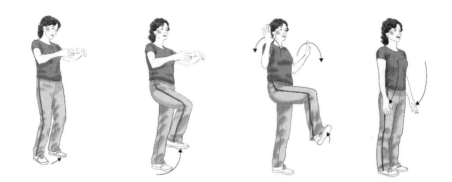

1. From the starting position, shift your weight onto your left foot.

2. Lift your hands to chest height as though you were holding a large balloon.

3. Breathe in.

4. Carefully raise your right leg until your knee is parallel to your hips.

5. If you think you might fall over, keep a chair close by. Just don't rest your weight on it.

6. Turn your palms outward. Extend your right foot forward slightly and tilt the sole of your foot out, as though pushing against a wall.

7. Breathe out and hold for 1 second.

8. Lower your foot and bring your arms down to your sides.

9. Repeat 10 to 30 times, alternating feet.

Pilates The hundred

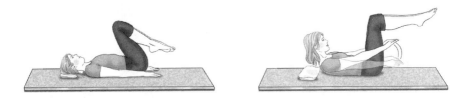

1. Lie on your back and draw your knees in toward your chest. Make sure your entire spine touches the mat.

2. Engage your powerhouse and bring your head and shoulders up.

3. Lift your feet up so your toes are just above knee level.

4. Lift your arms until they are parallel with the floor.

5. Pump your arms up and down, keeping them straight and stretched. Pump 5 times while you breathe in, and 5 times as you breathe out.

6. See if you can make it to 50 pumps without stopping. Eventually you should work up to 100 pumps.

Pilates Roll down

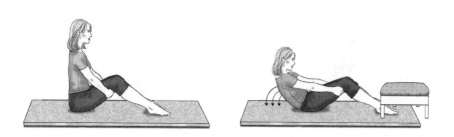

1. Sit up, with your back straight, and your legs slightly bent and hip-width apart.

   Make sure the soles of your feet touch the mat.

2. Wrap your hands under your thighs, close to your knees. Keep your shoulders down and your elbows pointed out like wings.

3. Tighten your buttocks and curve in your abdomen. Slowly lower your back down to the mat.

4. Imagine curling one vertebra down at a time. Keep your back and buttocks in a soft "c" curve.

5. As you roll, tuck your chin down and look at your abdomen.

6. Roll down as far as you can without letting go of your thighs. You may want to tuck your feet under a stool.

7. Hold for 3 deep breaths, then lift up gradually until you are back in a seated position.

8. Repeat 3 times.

Pilates Single leg stretch

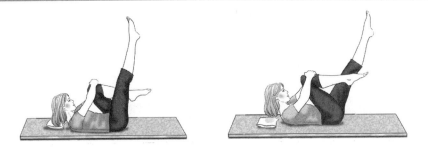

1. Lie on your back, with both knees pulled up to your chest.

2. Lift up and, with both hands, gently hug your left knee toward your shoulder. Keep your elbows pointed out like wings.

3. Point your right leg toward the ceiling.

4. Smoothly switch legs and repeat on the other side. Make sure your hips don't swivel but stay firmly against the mat.

5. Repeat 5 to 8 times.

Pilates Single leg circle

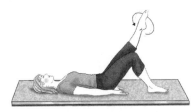

1. Lie flat on your mat, with your arms pressed down at your sides.

2. Bend one knee and point your other leg up at the ceiling.

3. Use your leg like a paintbrush. Pretend to paint circles on the ceiling.

4. Make sure your active hip stays firmly against the mat.

5. Circle 5 times clockwise, then 5 times counter-clockwise. Switch legs and repeat.

Pilates Spine stretch forward

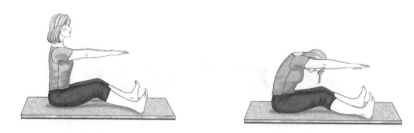

1. Sit straight and tall, with your legs softly bent and about hip-width apart. Point your toes up, as if your feet are pushing against a wall.

2. Hold your arms out straight in front of you at shoulder height.

3. As you exhale, pretend to dive between your arms. Lower your head, and tighten your stomach muscles.

4. Keep your lower back stationary and round your upper back.

5. Stretch forward, as if trying to reach the far wall.

6. Uncurl as you inhale, returning to your original upright position.

7. Repeat 3 to 5 times.

The Next Defense

When diet and exercise are not enough

Quick way to raise low blood sugar

You may be plagued by episodes of hypoglycemia, or low blood sugar, if you take insulin for diabetes. You'll recognize it by symptoms like sweating, shaking, tingling lips, fatigue, irritability, and poor coordination. It can happen anytime you don't eat enough, take too much insulin, or over-exercise. And when it does, your blood sugar level can drop below 70 milligrams per deciliter (mg/dl), knocking you out, putting you in a coma, or worse.

The next time you suffer from low blood sugar don't reach for candy, soda, or juice. Try glucose tablets or gels instead. They're more effective in raising your blood sugar and more nutritious. Here are some benefits.

Speed to your bloodstream. Glucose products are just that – pure glucose – and glucose is the Jesse Owens of the sugar world. In a race to get into your bloodstream, it's the fastest. That's what you want when you're in a fix with low blood sugar.

Candy, honey, and other everyday sources contain a mix of sugars and sometimes fat. This means they take longer to get into your system and raise your blood sugar than glucose does. Even ordinary table sugar works only half as well as pure glucose. Besides, many candies contain enough fat to shoot their calorie count through the roof – up to four times more than a glucose product.

You also should not eat diabetic snack bars or meal bars, like Extend Bar or Nite Bite, if you have an episode of low blood sugar. These bars are made to prevent low blood sugar, and they act too slowly.

Available in just the right dose. Experts recommend eating a quick 15 grams of carbohydrates when your blood sugar level falls below 70 mg/dl. Give your body another 15-gram dose if you're still hypoglycemic 15 to 20 minutes later.

Drugs that cause diabetes

Some drugs that help control your blood pressure may increase your risk for diabetes. Common prescription drugs that may actually cause type 2 diabetes include diuretics and beta blockers. Are you unknowingly taking them? Ask your doctor if other options, such as ACE inhibitors or angiotensin receptor blockers, would be safer.

Keep in mind the benefits of these diuretics and beta blockers may outweigh the risks, especially for people with certain risk factors. Never stop taking a drug your doctor prescribed without his approval. But, regardless of which blood pressure medication you take, be sure to ask your doctor to test you for high blood sugar at least once a year.

How can you tell if you're getting that exact dose with a chocolate bar or piece of hard candy? You can't. But glucose gels and tablets come in set doses, so you can be sure of the correct amount of carbohydrates. They vary by product, however, so read all labels carefully.

Easy on your wallet. For all of these benefits, you might expect these emergency glucose products to be pricey. On the contrary, three glucose tablets – enough to ward off a mild hypoglycemic attack – costs about 35 cents.

Convenient to keep on hand. So squirrel away supplies of glucose tablets in your pocketbook, in your car, and at home. Keep some with you at all times.

If you run out of glucose tablets, you can get by with more traditional remedies for low blood sugar, like syrup, honey, nondiet soda, hard candies, crackers, juice, sugar cubes, or gel cake frosting. Just be sure your sugar source is easy to use in case of an emergency and small enough to carry with you wherever you go.

Whatever you use, always be careful not to give food or glucose products to someone who has passed out. Instead, either give them a shot of glucagon or take them straight to the emergency room. If you don't have glucagon, on the way to the hospital, try putting some cake decorating gel or glucose gel inside their cheek and rubbing it from the outside until it dissolves.

New drugs to the rescue

When watching your diet and exercising more aren't enough to control type 2 diabetes, doctors often turn to drugs. Unfortunately, some drugs, including insulin and thiazolidinediones − Actos and Avandia − can cause significant weight gain. Excess weight tends to make diabetes worse. But now, several new drugs to control blood sugar have the added bonus of helping you lose weight.

Exenatide (Byetta). This injectable drug helps control blood sugar for people with type 2 diabetes. Although it is injected twice a day using a pre-filled pen, people seem to prefer it to other diabetes drugs. Why? This new drug, approved by the Food and Drug Administration (FDA) in 2005, promotes digestion and insulin production. People taking Byetta say it also works like an appetite suppressant. They eat less, which makes them shed pounds.

In one study, people taking Byetta lost an average of 5 pounds in six months, while another study found people lost 12 pounds in two years. What's more, the longer people take Byetta, the more weight they lose. Byetta is expensive at about $170 a month, but most health insurance companies cover it. Some people experience side effects like nausea, rashes, and fever, but they often diminish over time.

Sitagliptin (Januvia). This pill, approved by the FDA in 2006, helps keep blood sugar under control. Tests show it controls blood sugar as well as an older drug, glipizide (Glucotrol), but with less chance of excessively low blood sugar. In fact, Januvia is different from other diabetes drugs, acting both to encourage the pancreas to produce more insulin and to keep the liver from making more glucose. That's a double dose of blood sugar control.

People with diabetes may not like the high cost of Januvia – $90 to $180 per month. But they like the fact that it doesn't cause weight gain, like some older diabetes drugs.

Vildagliptin (Galvus). Researchers are working on yet another option to control blood sugar and aid in weight loss. This drug is currently being tested and awaiting FDA approval. Like Januvia, Galvus is a member of the class of drugs called DPP-IV inhibitors, which help your body handle glucose better. A once-a-day pill, Galvus controls blood sugar better than some of the traditional drugs, and it helps people with diabetes lose weight. This new drug seems to work even better in people who are elderly or obese.

Say good-bye to finger pricks

The days of needles and finger-pricking blood sugar monitors may be numbered. The FDA has approved GlucoWatch, a wristband monitor that uses tiny electrical charges to help measure blood sugar in the fluid between skin cells.

And now scientists say they have a contact lens that can measure the blood sugar in your tears. And you don't even have to cry to get results. Although the lens isn't available yet, stay tuned. It could be the next big thing you hear about in blood sugar monitoring.

Secrets to finding free or low-cost drugs

Believe it or not, you could qualify for free medication even if you're under age 65. In fact, some people with insurance or Medicare Part D still get help with their drug costs. Find out about the variety of options that could ease the hardship of paying for your prescription drugs.

Discover free medication programs. Drug companies offer Patient Assistance Programs (PAPs) to help people living on low incomes get free medication. You're most likely to qualify if you are ineligible for other assistance programs.

Plan to apply separately for each medication you take and be ready to provide proof-of-income documents. Your doctor or another health professional must also fill out forms on your behalf, so be prepared. And don't hesitate to fill prescriptions you'll use soon. It could take several weeks to find out if you qualify.

You may have heard you won't qualify for assistance if you enroll in Medicare Part D. But some programs have declared Part D participants eligible again. Regardless of whether you're enrolled in Part D or not, contact these organizations to find programs you might qualify for.

▸ Partnership for Prescription Assistance (PPA). Call toll-free 888-477-2669 or visit *www.pparx.org*. You'll find plenty of drug company PAPs and other programs for free or low-cost drugs.

▸ BenefitsCheckUp. Visit *www.benefitscheckup.org* if you're 55 or older. Learn which programs you qualify for if you don't have Medicare Part D.

▸ If you have Part D, how would you like to pay only $5 per prescription – no premiums, no deductibles? Find out if you qualify for the amazing "Extra Help" program by visiting *www.benefitscheckup.org*.

▶ RxAssist.org. Call 401-729-3284 or visit *www.rxassist.org*. You must register for a free account to use the site.

▶ NeedyMeds.com. Visit *www.needymeds.com* or call 215-625-9609. You'll find drug company PAPs plus government programs, discount drug cards, and generic drug assistance.

▶ Together Rx Access. Apply for the Together Rx Access drug discount card for up to 40 percent off medications from several big-name drug companies. To qualify, you must meet income requirements, be ineligible for Medicare, and have no prescription drug coverage. Call 800-444-4106 or visit *www.togetherrxaccess.com*.

▶ The Medicine Program. If your medication costs are a financial hardship and you lack drug coverage, you could qualify for assistance regardless of age even if you earn $60,000 a year. Visit *www.themedicineprogram.com* or call 573-996-7300. Although you must pay a $5 processing fee, the money is refundable if you do not receive drug payment help. Don't confuse The Medicine Program with My Free Medicine. My Free Medicine is a fraudulent program that charges for patient assistance application forms. You can get these forms free from Partnership for Prescription Assistance and other sources.

Cut insurance copays. If you have insurance, help is available for steep copayments that cause financial hardship.

▶ Patient Services, Inc. Get up to two years of copay assistance for selected illnesses and conditions. Call 800-366-7741 or visit *www.uneedpsi.org* for more information.

▶ Patient Advocate Foundation Co-Pay Relief. Call 866-512-3861 or visit *www.copays.org* to find out the medical and financial requirements for this program. You can qualify even if you have Medicare Part D.

Speedy test detects trouble early

New technology may make it possible to find out if you are on the road to diabetes — or to find diabetes complications if you already have the disease — by turning on a light. No fasting, no drawing blood, no problem.

Skin autofluorescence is light given off by cells based on certain changes when ultraviolet light hits them. It's used to measure the amount of toxins in the skin of people with diabetes. These toxins, called advanced glycation end products (AGEs), build up when blood sugar is too high.

High levels of AGEs in your skin mean you're suffering from damage to small blood vessels. This kind of microvascular injury can lead to kidney damage (nephropathy) or eye damage (retinopathy). Researchers can find your level of AGEs by holding a black light near your skin and checking to see how much light is emitted.

Similar technology is being developed to diagnose diabetes and prediabetes in people at risk of the disease. Traditionally, you'd have to have a blood test to see how high your fasting blood sugar level is. That means going without food overnight, then dragging yourself to a doctor in the morning to have blood drawn and tested.

But the new Scout light, being developed by VeraLight Inc., uses a light to measure the AGE levels in your skin. So far, it's more accurate than traditional blood sugar tests at identifying people with diabetes or prediabetes. The light test takes about a minute. The Scout machine is not yet available, but it's expected to be in doctors' offices soon.

Fight heart attack and stroke with aspirin

Discover the one-a-day, over-the-counter pill that could keep people with diabetes from having a deadly heart attack or stroke. Even better, it's not an expensive vitamin. It's plain old aspirin and it may help you in more ways than one.

Cardiovascular disease, which includes heart attack and stroke, is the leading cause of death in the United States. On top of that, having diabetes can double, triple, even quadruple your risk. That's why the American Diabetes Association recommends people over age 40 who have diabetes take a daily, low-dose aspirin (75 to 162 milligrams) to cut their risk of heart attack and stroke.

Experts think people with diabetes produce too much thromboxane, a chemical that narrows blood vessels and causes blood

High-tech way to monitor blood sugar

Your computer may be better than a doctor at helping you monitor your blood sugar. That's what researchers in Korea found in a lengthy study of people with type 2 diabetes.

The researchers followed 80 people struggling to control their blood sugar, dividing them into two groups. Those in one group tested their blood sugar as usual, then saw their doctors every three months for advice on keeping it stable.

People in the other group used an online monitoring program, reporting the results of their blood sugar tests into a chart on the Internet. They could also post questions online and get advice from health-care professionals. The people who used Internet monitoring fared much better. They had fewer dramatic changes in blood sugar, and their overall blood sugar levels were lower.

Some electronic blood sugar monitors offer online information management. Check the features before you purchase a monitor.

platelets to clump together. This can lead to blood clots and narrowed arteries. Aspirin keeps your body from using thromboxane and makes platelets slippery so they don't stick together.

Aspirin in small, regular doses helps prevent blood clots from forming, which reduces your risk of heart attack and stroke. For people with diabetes, aspirin also helps by warding off diabetic retinopathy, which can result in blindness.

Unfortunately, most people who could benefit from aspirin therapy aren't using it. Even though researchers have known for a long time about the benefits of aspirin therapy for diabetics, only about 12 percent of people with diabetes take aspirin regularly. Many others opt for treatment with fancier, more expensive statin drugs. But studies show aspirin reduces heart disease risk as well as statins at a fraction of the cost.

Recent studies on overweight mice also showed that aspirin in extremely high doses reversed some signs of type 2 diabetes and reduced low-grade inflammation, which is linked to insulin resistance. The high doses of aspirin used in the study effectively reversed diabetes in the mice. Researchers are now investigating how this high-dose aspirin therapy might work on people. Unfortunately, aspirin in high doses can cause intestinal bleeding and harm your liver and kidneys.

For now, ask your doctor if you should try daily, low-dose aspirin therapy to reduce your risk of heart attack and stroke. Aspirin therapy is not right for everyone, especially people who bleed easily, have liver disease, or take blood-thinning medications. Talk with your doctor before trying it.

Surprise benefit from a cholesterol-lowering drug

It's like getting three drugs for the price of one. Bezofibrate is a cholesterol-lowering drug that also cuts your risk of stroke. And now, researchers have learned it might reduce your risk of type 2 diabetes, too.

In a study in Israel, scientists compared two groups of people with prediabetes – one group of men who took bezofibrate and another that took a placebo. They discovered that the bezofibrate group was 30 percent less likely to get diabetes than the placebo group.

Moreover, people in the placebo group developed diabetes earlier than men in the bezofibrate group. Bezofibrate might delay diabetes as well as reduce your risk of getting it at all.

Although bezofibrate isn't available in the United States, other heart-related drugs have also shown promise against diabetes. If you have prediabetes and already take medication for heart disease or high blood pressure, ask your doctor whether your medication helps prevent diabetes. If it doesn't, your doctor can help you decide whether switching to another medicine is right for you.

Guide to safer, more effective supplements

Your best defense against unsafe supplements and phony therapies is to be a smart consumer. Learn the facts backing a product or treatment, get trustworthy advice, and complain if you think you've been taken for a ride.

Know what you're getting. You can't always count on a supplement's label to tell you what it contains. The independent laboratory ConsumerLab.com tests health and nutrition products for quality and safety. They publish their results on their Web site, *www.ConsumerLab.com.*

Here you can find out which supplement brands had the right amount of active ingredients, which did not, and which posed health hazards. You can read partial results from their tests for free, but to see the full reports, you must subscribe to their service the way you would a magazine.

Get more from your medicine

About 40 to 50 percent of people with diabetes don't take their medicine correctly. Follow instructions on the package carefully. If there's anything you don't understand, call your doctor or pharmacist.

Heed the latest warnings. The Food and Drug Administration (FDA) issues warnings about supplements as soon as they learn of potential dangers. To stay up to date, visit their Web site at *www.cfsan.fda.gov* and click on "Dietary Supplements," or call the FDA's toll-free information line 888-463-6332.

ConsumerLab.com also publishes recalls, warnings, and other alerts on their Web site. You can read the latest alert for free, but you must subscribe to their service to see old ones.

Sometimes the FDA and Federal Trade Commission (FTC) take legal action against sellers, especially those who lie about the healing powers or safety of their product. Find out who's guilty at *www.ftc.gov* or *www.fda.gov/oc/enforcement.html.*

Talk to your personal expert. Considering a supplement or alternative therapy? Run it past your doctor. She can warn you about the dangers, help you watch for side effects, and avoid prescribing medicine that could interact with your supplements.

Report supplement dangers. The FDA collects complaints about supplement side effects and uses them to build a case against dangerous products. You or your doctor should report supplement-related side effects to the FDA by calling 1-800-332-1088 or filling out a form online at *www.fda.gov/medwatch.*

Filter out the hype. Too often, sellers exaggerate the benefits of their products. Find out for yourself what hard science says about an alternative treatment. Look for these reliable books at your local library.

▸ *Tyler's Honest Herbal* by Steven Foster and Varro Tyler

▸ *Botanical Medicines* by Dennis J. McKenna, Kenneth Jones, and Kerry Hughes

▸ *Alternative Medicine: The Definitive Guide*, 2nd edition, by Burton Goldberg, John W. Anderson, and Larry Trivieri

A few Web sites offer easy-to-read, unbiased information about herbs, nutrition, and alternative treatments. For instance, the Office of Dietary Supplements, a department of the National Institutes of Health (NIH), provides information about supplement safety and side effects. Visit their Web site at *dietary-supplements.info.nih.gov* and click on "Health Information." Check out these resources for additional advice.

▸ National Center for Complementary and Alternative Medicine at *www.nccam.nih.gov*

▸ MayoClinic.com at *www.mayoclinic.com*

Foil heart disease with fish oil

If you have high triglycerides, stop turning your liver into a fat factory that could threaten your heart. Take this supplement to "oil" your liver's machinery and make it work right

Get the lowdown on triglycerides. You already know that people with diabetes have a higher risk of heart disease than average. You should also know that a high triglyceride level in your blood is a pretty powerful indicator of heart disease risk.

Triglycerides come from the fats in food you eat and from excess carbohydrates. Many health experts think fish oil interferes with your liver's ability to change the carbohydrates into triglycerides. And that could help you get triglycerides back under control.

Say sayonara to fish oil fears. For some time, experts were concerned fish oil raised blood sugar levels. However, when they took another look at more than a dozen studies, following over 800 people with diabetes, they realized this just wasn't so. Researchers noted fish oil caused no significant increase in blood sugar.

Supplementing with fish oil is one way to get two important omega-3 fatty acids – eicosapentaenoic acid (EPA) and docosahexaenoic acid (DHA). Studies by two consumer organizations show that most fish oil supplements contain the EPA and DHA amounts claimed on the label and are free of contaminants.

Seek expert advice. Although the American Heart Association has recommended 2 to 4 grams of omega-3 fatty acids daily to control triglycerides, talk with your doctor before you take any amount of fish oil supplements. These supplements may not be safe for people with some health conditions or those who take certain medications or herbs.

For example, fish oil capsules might thin your blood too much if you take them with blood thinners, like Coumadin (warfarin), or NSAIDs, like ibuprofen and aspirin. Very high doses of omega-3s can also increase bleeding time and may suppress the immune system.

Avoid distressing side effects. If your doctor approves the use of fish oil supplements, don't start on the full dose right away. That can cause side effects like gas, burping, and fishy aftertaste. Instead, start at a low dose and make gradual increases to the recommended amount.

Super antioxidant stymies pain

ALA or alpha-lipoic acid, found only in tiny amounts in food, makes a big impact on diabetes. It's best known for improving symptoms of diabetic polyneuropathy, a common complication of diabetes that includes painful nerve damage in your feet, legs, and hands. And studies show it can also boost insulin sensitivity.

Unlike most antioxidants, alpha-lipoic acid works in both fat and water. That, in itself, would be enough to earn a spot on the antioxidant all-star team. But this antioxidant doesn't hog all the glory. Like the best athletes, alpha-lipoic acid also makes its teammates better.

That's because it recycles other antioxidants to make them more effective. When using antioxidants such as vitamins C and E, it's important to also take this little-known coenzyme. It keeps them working at maximum speed, improving sugar metabolism up to 50 percent. The result – a winning team in the fight against diabetes.

Along with its fellow antioxidants, alpha-lipoic acid battles oxidative stress, a major factor in diabetic complications. Alpha-lipoic acid also improves microcirculation, or blood flow in the very small blood vessels.

Several studies, mostly from Germany, support the use of alpha-lipoic acid for diabetes. In fact, Germans have been using alpha-lipoic acid to treat polyneuropathy for more than 30 years.

▶ Studies indicate that taking 600 milligrams (mg) of alpha-lipoic acid, also known as thioctic acid, intravenously for three weeks improves symptoms of neuropathy.

▶ A small German study showed that taking 1,800 mg of alpha-lipoic acid per day orally for three weeks also helped with symptoms of neuropathy.

▶ Another German study found that oral alpha-lipoic acid improved insulin sensitivity compared to placebo.

▶ A Croatian study determined that high doses of alpha-lipoic acid may improve nerve function in people with diabetic polyneuropathy.

The most common dosages are 600 mg per day when taken intravenously and 800 mg to 1,800 mg per day when taken orally. Safety does not seem to be an issue. Alpha-lipoic acid has one drawback — it doesn't stay in your bloodstream very long. That's why intravenous alpha-lipoic acid seems more effective than the oral variety. But taking supplements intravenously is not practical, or desirable, for the average person.

This problem might be remedied in the future. Taking enteric-coated capsules, which dissolve in your intestines instead of your stomach, or those with a time-released formula might help make alpha-lipoic acid more effective. Keep your eyes open for these products.

Right now, alpha-lipoic acid looks like a star-in-waiting, sort of like an elite minor league prospect. But it needs more conclusive long-term studies before it can be recommended without reservations. Talk with your doctor before taking supplemental alpha-lipoic acid, which may interact with other drugs or supplements designed to do the same thing.

Douse inflammation with herbs

Inflammation can be a hidden factor in diabetes and many of its complications. But you can tap into the healing power of herbs to help. Just be sure to first get the facts about herbs that work and ones to steer clear of.

Before you use an herbal supplement, talk to your doctor. Some herbs are dangerous for people with certain health conditions, and others don't mix well with drugs. In fact, many herbs in the following table interact with drugs used for heart conditions and other illnesses people with diabetes are more likely to have. The herb-drug combinations listed in the box on the next page are good examples.

Beware dangerous herb-drug combos

Watch out for the following herb-drug pairings.

▸ St. John's wort weakens the power of several prescription drugs, including digoxin, warfarin, cyclosporine, antibiotics, sedatives, birth control pills, cholesterol-lowering drugs, antipsychotics, theophylline, and protease inhibitors.

▸ Garlic, ginkgo, vitamin E, and papaya are natural blood-thinners that prevent blood from clotting. When combined with blood-thinning drugs, like warfarin or aspirin, they could cause dangerous internal bleeding.

▸ Yohimbine is an herb used for impotence, but it can boost your risk for high blood pressure when taken with tricyclic antidepressants.

▸ Combining ginseng with the MAO inhibitor phenelzine may lead to mania in depressed people.

▸ In rare cases, fish oil, borage oil, and evening primrose oil could trigger bruising and nosebleeds if taken with aspirin or other NSAIDs, such as ibuprofen or naproxen.

If you're scheduled for surgery, stop taking all supplements three weeks ahead of time. They can cause complications such as bleeding, heart instability, low blood sugar, and blood pressure changes.

What's more, many of these herbs could also lower your blood sugar and cause hypoglycemia, especially if you take them with drugs or supplements that also lower blood sugar. Fortunately, your doctor can help you figure out which of these herbs are safe for you.

She may also be able to recommend the best dosage and how often you should take it.

Be aware that some herbs have a stronger reputation than others. The effectiveness ratings in the table on page 353 can help you tell which herbs are known powerhouses and which ones need more testing. The ratings are based on how much research has been done on the herbs as treatments for each condition or symptom.

*** – Remedy has strong scientific evidence it works.

** – Remedy has weak scientific evidence it works.

* – Traditional remedy has little scientific evidence.

Now you're ready to use the table on the following page to help you fight the inflammation behind diabetes and its complications. Choose from among 13 inflammation-fighting herbs and spices ready to do battle against heart disease, arthritis, diabetes, and more.

For detailed information about a particular herb, see the list of herb and drug interactions at the U.S. government's Web site, *www.medlineplus.gov*. Select "Drugs & Supplements," then find your desired herb in the alphabetical list.

Take the Oriental root to better health

This popular Asian remedy and all-healing herb is revealed to the West at last. It's called ginseng, and it could help improve your health in several ways.

Regulates your blood sugar. For decades, ginseng's main active ingredients, ginsenosides, have been isolated from the ginseng root to treat the high blood sugar of diabetes. Ginsenosides from both the American ginseng and the Asian ginseng plant can help balance blood sugar levels and increase the amount of insulin in the blood. Repeated, high-quality research has tested the effects in numerous

Herb	Condition or symptom	Effectiveness rating	May cause hypoglycemia
alfalfa	diabetes	**	Yes
	heart disease	**	
	inflammation	*	
bromelain	inflammation	***	Unlikely
	rheumatoid arthritis	**	
chamomile	insomnia	**	Yes
	skin inflammation	**	
dandelion	diabetes	**	Yes
	inflammation	**	
devil's claw	back pain	***	Yes
	inflammation	*	
	osteoarthritis	***	
elder	inflammation	*	Yes
eyebright	inflammation	**	Yes
feverfew	inflammation	*	Unlikely
	migraine headaches	***	
	rheumatoid arthritis	**	
ginseng	diabetes	***	Yes
	inflammation	*	
goldenseal	inflammation	*	Unlikely
lavender	anxiety	***	Unlikely
	inflammation	*	
St. John's wort	depression (mild to moderate)	***	Yes
	inflammation	*	
turmeric	diabetes	*	Unlikely
	inflammation	**	
	osteoarthritis	**	

studies. The research suggests it may cut both fasting and after-meal blood sugar levels, plus lower your three-month average levels.

Protects your heart and blood vessels. Ginseng unleashes antioxidants, which can fight free radicals that damage your arteries. Ginseng also jumps in to prevent platelets from ganging up into clots that can cause heart attacks.

This powerful little root might even fight high cholesterol. Some herbal experts think ginsenosides help your liver snatch up cholesterol particles before they can wreak havoc in your bloodstream.

Although past studies suggest ginseng helps control cholesterol, results from animal research have been mixed. But recently, a study found that eight male college students lowered total cholesterol, harmful LDL cholesterol, and triglycerides after taking ginseng extract for just eight weeks. In addition, their levels of heart-helping HDL cholesterol rose. More research is needed to verify the study's results, to find out whether ginseng can work safely for everyone, and to see how long it might control cholesterol.

Prevents diabetic vision loss and more. Ginseng also appears to be a powerful antioxidant that could prevent diabetic vision loss and kidney complications by protecting delicate blood vessels from oxidative damage. It could also lessen stress, relieve fatigue, improve memory, and increase your strength.

If you decide to take ginseng supplements, check with your doctor first. Mild side effects can include nausea, diarrhea, insomnia, headaches, or low blood pressure. Here are some serious side effects to keep in mind.

▶ If you have high blood pressure or low blood sugar, this herb might make your problems worse. Ginseng can drive blood pressure up or blood sugar down. It can also make trouble by teaming up with insulin or drugs that reduce blood sugar.

Choose a better blood sugar monitor

A good glucose monitor for home use can really help keep your blood sugar under control. Consider features like these before you buy.

▶ Check which products your insurance company covers. Also, remember that the cost of test strips, which you need each time you test and are specific to each monitor, will probably be higher than the cost of the machine over time. Factor that difference into your choice.

▶ A number of monitors calibrate themselves, while others require extra steps.

▶ The new monitors are small, light, and portable. "Test drive" a few models to see how comfortable they feel in your hand and whether the screen is easy to read. Also, check how much blood is needed and how long you must wait for results.

▶ Some monitors let you test blood drawn from sites other than your fingertips. Ask your doctor if it's right for you.

▶ Women with a history of breast cancer should avoid ginseng since it may stimulate breast cancer cells to grow.

▶ Ginseng interacts with a long list of supplements and prescription drugs. For example, don't use ginseng if you are taking warfarin (Coumadin), phenelzine (Nardil), or nifedipine. Also, don't take ginseng with large amounts of caffeine or other stimulants. Talk to your doctor or pharmacist to find out if ginseng interacts with a medicine you take.

Before you buy ginseng supplements, read the label carefully. *Panax ginseng* – also called Asian ginseng – is one of the "true" ginsengs, not an imitator often passed off for the real thing. It's also the most well-researched. American ginseng or *Panax quinquefolius L.* is generally considered milder than Asian ginseng.

Recently, a major consumer organization tested 18 brands of ginseng supplements. Only one harbored contaminants, but another failed to match the potency claimed on its label. To avoid these problems, look for ginseng supplements that feature the Consumer Labs Seal of Approved Quality on the container.

Also, look for an extract labeled "standardized" that contains at least 3 percent total ginsenosides – or 30 milligrams (mg) per gram. Experts usually recommend taking 200 milligrams.

Latest buzz on promising weight-loss pill

The popular supplement CLA stands for "conjugated linoleic acid," but it could just as well stand for "conquer large abdomens."

This easy-to-find pill claims to banish the most dangerous kind of fat – abdominal fat or the fat around your middle – and helps you keep weight off once you lose it. Could CLA be the next great breakthrough in the battle of the bulge?

Examine the evidence. Recent studies suggest CLA, a natural fatty acid, may help with weight control. University of Wisconsin professor Michael Pariza, Ph.D., led a six-month study of 80 overweight people. They dieted, exercised, and lost weight. When they stopped their diets, however, many people regained some of the weight they had lost.

Those who did not take CLA added pounds at a typical ratio of 75 percent fat to 25 percent muscle. But for the people taking CLA, the results were pleasantly different.

"The ratio was more like 50:50 — 50 percent fat and 50 percent muscle," Pariza says. "That is very significant. It leads to the idea that CLA could be useful in weight management. Our results also showed that CLA made it easier for people to stay on their diets."

Pariza's study isn't the only one that gives dieters hope. Two smaller studies also support CLA. A four-week Swedish study of 25 people found that CLA decreases abdominal fat. And a 12-week Norwegian study of 47 people showed CLA reduces body fat. In all three studies, people took about 3 to 4 grams of CLA a day.

Wait and see. While CLA seems generally safe, more studies are needed. For example, no one knows the long-term effects of taking CLA.

No one knows for sure that it works, either. CLA produced all sorts of amazing results in animal studies, but not all human studies

Save big on a new prescription

Drug companies constantly shower doctors with free samples of prescription drugs to hand out to patients like you. So don't hesitate to ask your doctor for free drug samples anytime she writes a prescription for a new drug. Samples can save you money in ways you might not expect.

For example, you'll have time to comparison shop for the best prices until your samples run out. Finding the cheapest source for your medicine could lead to years of savings. Moreover, prescription drug samples are a golden opportunity to road test a drug that is new to you. You won't lose a dime if the drug causes unbearable side effects or turns out to be ineffective.

showed the same effects. It might depend on what form of CLA you take – and you can't always tell what form you're getting by reading the supplement's label.

Consider the cons. Possible side effects include nausea, upset stomach, and fatigue. To combat nausea, some experts recommend taking CLA with milk. While some experts claim CLA may improve insulin levels, others do not recommend it for people with type 2 diabetes, liver disease, or insulin resistance. In fact, recent research shows CLA may actually raise blood sugar levels and make your body even more resistant to insulin. If you have diabetes, that's exactly what you don't want to have happen.

CLA is a natural ingredient in whole foods such as beef, dairy products, poultry, and eggs. But you'd have to eat an awful lot of these foods to match the amount you get in a supplement – and that wouldn't exactly help you lose weight.

Remember, CLA is not a miracle pill. It seems promising, but it's not 100 percent proven yet. Before you start popping "magic" pills, ask your doctor about CLA.

New 'whey' to battle blood sugar

Little Miss Muppet may have had the right idea when she was digging into those curds and whey. Recent research found that adding whey protein powder to meals can help fight high blood sugar.

In the study, people who normally controlled their diabetes with diet ate four meals designed to make blood sugar rise quickly. The researchers added whey protein powder mixed in a drink to one breakfast and one lunch, while the other breakfast and lunch included a placebo.

Blood tests showed that the participants made more insulin after eating their meals with whey. Their blood sugar levels were also lower after the whey-laced lunch than after the lunch with placebo.

But, oddly enough, whey protein powder didn't lower blood sugar after breakfast. The scientists think whey may be more effective at lunch than at breakfast because insulin resistance is often higher in the morning.

This study was small and more research is needed to know whether whey protein powder really works. Moreover, whey protein may not be a good choice for people who are lactose intolerant or have milk allergies. But if you'd like to try whey powder, talk with your doctor. He can tell you whether whey protein might be right for you.

You may also want to ask him whether you can safely eat more low-fat dairy products. Dairy foods and drinks often contain whey, and they've been shown to lower women's odds of getting diabetes. Although nobody knows for sure whether dairy helps people with type 2 diabetes, at least one study suggests it might. So get your doctor's advice on how much dairy you can safely eat and which dairy foods and beverages are best for your health.

Discover the benefits of fenugreek

You've tasted it in curry — now taste this superb spice again, and see why people with diabetes are giving fenugreek a closer look. A bitter-tasting legume, it's been used for thousands of years in Asia, Africa, and parts of Europe to treat a variety of ailments — to settle a gassy stomach, improve appetite, and soothe inflamed skin. Now Western medicine suspects fenugreek may help people with diabetes in two important ways.

When people with mild, type 2 diabetes took fenugreek, their blood sugar levels fell significantly. It's important to note that healthy people saw no change, and people with severe diabetes experienced only a slight decrease. Animal studies suggest taking fenugreek every day might lower total and LDL (bad) cholesterol.

Travel tips to keep medication safe

Don't leave insulin, other drugs, and testing strips in a hot car, and don't pack them in a suitcase to be checked on an airplane. Too much heat or cold can damage drugs, especially liquids. It can also harm testing strips. Carry your fragile supplies in an insulated bag, and never leave it in a hot car.

Health professionals say they need more evidence before they can recommend fenugreek as a weapon against high blood sugar and cholesterol. In fact, experts aren't sure exactly how fenugreek lowers blood sugar and cholesterol, but they think its soluble fiber and plant steroids, called saponins, may play a role.

You can buy fenugreek at many natural foods stores and at markets that specialize in foods from India. People with diabetes in the study took about one-half teaspoon (2.5 grams) of fenugreek powder twice a day for three months to get these health-saving results.

Be sure to talk to your doctor before trying fenugreek. Fenugreek may interact with medications for blood sugar or heart-related problems. You also shouldn't take fenugreek if you are allergic to chickpeas, because you might be allergic to fenugreek as well.

If your doctor gives you the green light to take fenugreek, be sure to monitor your blood sugar regularly. Fenugreek could push your blood sugar too low, especially if you're already taking diabetes drugs or making lifestyle changes to reduce your blood sugar.

Get the facts about chromium

Many people have taken a shine to chromium. But before you shell out money for this popular pill, check out the theory behind chromium's success – and the evidence that supports it.

Chromium is a trace mineral found naturally in plants, animals, and soil. You can also find it in supplement form as chromium picolinate, which is easier for your body to absorb. This is especially handy for people with diabetes who need more chromium but have a harder time converting it to a usable form.

Chromium helps regulate glucose, or blood sugar, by increasing the action of insulin. Experts theorize that chromium teams up with a protein called low molecular weight chromium-binding substance (LMWCr) to kick-start the insulin receptor. In a domino effect, this prompts the cellular signaling mechanism to do its job and let glucose into the cells.

Perhaps the strongest evidence for chromium comes from Dr. Richard Anderson's 1997 study that showed chromium picolinate reduced glucose and insulin concentrations in people with type 2 diabetes in China.

For four months, the 180 people in the study received either a placebo or chromium picolinate. One supplement group took 200 micrograms (mcg) of chromium picolinate a day, while the other took 1,000 mcg a day.

Both supplement groups significantly decreased their insulin levels and their glycosylated hemoglobin, a sign of high blood sugar. Those in the higher dose group also slashed their glucose levels.

But people in the study weighed an average of only 152 pounds, and their dietary intake of chromium before the study was not measured. That might explain why other studies have been inconclusive.

While taking chromium supplements for diabetes seems promising, reviews by the FDA and the American Diabetes Association say there is not enough solid evidence to recommend it.

If you choose to supplement your diet with chromium, experts say aim for at least 200 mcg a day. Some health professionals even recommend taking as much as 1,000 mcg a day. Keep in mind this far exceeds the Institute of Medicine's Adequate Intake of 20 mcg a day for women over age 50 and 30 mcg a day for men over age 50. Although chromium seems safe, there is a lack of information about the long-term effects of chromium supplementation, especially at high doses.

Of some concern is a recent University of Alabama study that found chromium picolinate causes DNA damage in fruit flies. Similar findings have been reported in studies of rats. While this does not necessarily translate into danger for humans, the possibility of danger remains.

Talk with your doctor before taking chromium supplements for diabetes. It can interact with both prescription and over-the-counter medications. For example, it might change or lower the amount of medication you need, particularly if you're taking drugs to control blood sugar.

Chromium may even increase your blood sugar if you're already taking corticosteroids. Also, don't forget that people with certain health conditions — such as depression, bipolar disorder, or a suppressed immune system — shouldn't take chromium supplements.

2 ways to slash health care costs

You might get medical treatments for a fraction of the cost or even free. Here's how to find out if you qualify.

Discover your options. If you are 55 or older, use a computer at your home or local library to visit *www.benefitscheckup.org* on the

How to get free medical advice

Know where to go online to get free help from top medical institutions 24 hours a day.

▶ Mayo Clinic. Learn from one of the world's most respected clinics. This site features information on health conditions, drugs, and more. Go to *www.mayoclinic.com*.

▶ InteliHealth. Get the benefit of an Ivy League education from this site, featuring information from Harvard Medical School. Learn at *www.intelihealth.com*.

▶ Drug InfoNet. Read all about prescription drugs at this useful site, which also provides information and links to other sites on a variety of topics. Disease information, government sites, hospitals, medical schools, health news — get it all at *www.druginfonet.com*.

▶ WebMD. Get information on any illness at this superb site. Just pay a visit to *www.webmd.com*.

And, of course, it's always a good idea to check the health information from the American Diabetes Association at *www.diabetes.org*.

Internet. Click the "Find More Benefits Programs" option and then click the "Comprehensive" option. You'll fill out a questionnaire to help find benefits where you live. But rest assured, all the information will be kept confidential.

This electronic service is free. In about 30 minutes, you'll find out if any programs can save you money based on your specific needs. It's that simple.

Get help from Uncle Sam. A little-known government program could pay all your hospital care. Under the Hill-Burton program, the federal government says certain health facilities must give medical care away for free or at reduced costs. Here's why. In 1946, the government began giving money to some health care facilities. The hospitals, clinics, and nursing homes that get these funds must give something back in return — free or low-cost services to people in their communities.

Your eligibility is based on your income, but you don't have to be in the poorhouse to qualify. Hospitals, clinics, and other facilities may offer free or inexpensive services to people with an income up to twice the poverty level. This program won't, however, cover private doctor and private pharmacy charges.

Find out if you can take advantage of this windfall. Call the Hill-Burton hotline toll-free at 800-638-0742 for more details and a list of hospitals, clinics, nursing homes, and other facilities in your area that participate in this special program. You can apply before or after you receive care, even if your bill has gone to a collections agency.

Keep in mind that different facilities offer different services under Hill-Burton. Call or visit the facility and ask someone in the Admissions, Business, or Patient Accounts office about Hill-Burton assistance. They can tell you what services they offer and whether you qualify.

Index